Crisis Services

Editors

MARGARET E. BALFOUR
MATTHEW L. GOLDMAN

PSYCHIATRIC CLINICS OF NORTH AMERICA

www.psych.theclinics.com

Consulting Editor
HARSH K. TRIVEDI

September 2024 • Volume 47 • Number 3

ELSEVIER

1600 John F. Kennedy Boulevard • Suite 1800 • Philadelphia, Pennsylvania, 19103-2899

http://www.theclinics.com

PSYCHIATRIC CLINICS OF NORTH AMERICA Volume 47, Number 3
September 2024 ISSN 0193-953X, ISBN-13: 978-0-443-12909-4

Editor: Megan Ashdown
Developmental Editor: Varun Gopal

Psychiatric Clinics of North America (ISSN 0193-953X) is published quarterly by Elsevier Inc., 360 Park Avenue South, New York, NY 10010-1710. Months of issue are March, June, September, and December. Business and Editorial Offices: 1600 John F. Kennedy Blvd., Suite 1800, Philadelphia, PA 19103-2899. Periodicals postage paid at New York, NY and additional mailing offices. Subscription prices are $362.00 per year (US individuals), $100.00 per year (US students/residents), $422.00 per year (Canadian individuals), $535.00 per year (international individuals), and $220.00 per year (international students/residents), $100.00 per year (Canadian & students/residents). For institutional access pricing please contact Customer Service via the contact information below. Foreign air speed delivery is included in all *Clinics'* subscription prices. All prices are subject to change without notice. Orders, claims, and journal inquiries: Please visit our Support Hub page https://service.elsevier.com for assistance.

Reprints. For copies of 100 or more, of articles in this publication, please contact the Commercial Reprints Department, Elsevier Inc., 360 Park Avenue South, New York, New York 10010-1710. Tel.: 212-633-3874, Fax: 212-633-3820, E-mail: reprints@elsevier.com.

Psychiatric Clinics of North America is covered in *MEDLINE/PubMed (Index Medicus), Current Contents/Social and Behavioral Sciences, Social Science Citation Index, Embase/Excerpta Medica,* and PsycINFO.

Contributors

CONSULTING EDITOR

HARSH K. TRIVEDI, MD, MBA
President and CEO, Sheppard Pratt, Baltimore, Maryland

EDITORS

MARGARET E. BALFOUR, MD, PhD
Associate Professor, Department of Psychiatry, University of Arizona College of Medicine, Tucson, Arizona; Chief of Quality and Clinical Innovation, Connections Health Solutions, Phoenix, Arizona

MATTHEW L. GOLDMAN, MD, MS
Volunteer Clinical Assistant Professor, Department of Psychiatry and Behavioral Sciences, University of Washington; Medical Director, Crisis Care Centers Initiative, King County Department of Community and Human Services, Seattle, Washington

AUTHORS

CURTIS N. ADAMS, MD
Assistant Professor, Department of Psychiatry, University of Maryland School of Medicine, Baltimore, Maryland

LISA ANACKER, MD
Adjunct Clinical Professor, Department of Psychiatry, University of Michigan, Ann Arbor, Michigan; Staff Psychiatrist and Consulting Forensic Examiner, Center for Forensic Psychiatry, Saline, Michigan

MARGARET E. BALFOUR, MD, PhD
Associate Professor, Department of Psychiatry, University of Arizona College of Medicine, Tucson, Arizona; Chief of Quality and Clinical Innovation, Connections Health Solutions, Phoenix, Arizona

CHRIS A. CARSON, MD, MBA
Chief Strategy Officer, Connections Health Solutions, Phoenix, Arizona

ENRICO G. CASTILLO, MD, MS
Associate Professor and Associate Vice Chair for Justice, Equity, Diversity, and Inclusion, Department of Psychiatry, Center for Social Medicine, Jane and Terry Semel Institute for Neuroscience and Human Behavior, David Geffen School of Medicine, UCLA, Los Angeles, California

MICHAEL T. COMPTON, MD, MPH
Professor, Department of Psychiatry, Columbia University Vagelos College of Physicians and Surgeons, New York State Psychiatric Institute, New York, New York

ROBERT O. COTES, MD
Associate Professor, Department of Psychiatry and Behavioral Sciences, Emory University School of Medicine, Atlanta, Georgia

JOHN DRAPER, PhD
President of Research and Development, Behavioral Health Link, Inc, Brooklyn, New York

MATTHEW EDWARDS, MD
Assistant Professor, Psychiatry, Stanford University School of Medicine, Stanford, California

ASHLEY A. FOSTER, MD
Assistant Professor, Department of Emergency Medicine, University of California, San Francisco, San Francisco, California

ALEXIS FRENCH, PhD
Assistant Professor, Department of Psychiatry and Behavioral Sciences, Duke University, Durham, North Carolina

MATTHEW L. GOLDMAN, MD, MS
Volunteer Clinical Assistant Professor, Department of Psychiatry and Behavioral Sciences, University of Washington; Medical Director, Crisis Care Centers Initiative, King County Department of Community and Human Services, Seattle, Washington

ANN L. HACKMAN, MD
Assistant Professor, Department of Psychiatry, University of Maryland School of Medicine, Baltimore, Maryland

KEN HOPPER, MD, MBA
Assistant Dean of Health Systems Science Education, Alice L. Walton School of Medicine, Bentonville, Arkansas

NICOLE JACKSON, DSW, LCSW
Senior Associate, Lorio Forensics, Atlanta, Georgia

SAMUEL W. JACKSON, MD
Co-Director of Public Psychiatry Education at SUNY Downstate's Adult Psychiatry Residency Program, Department of Psychiatry, SUNY Downstate Health Sciences University, Brooklyn, New York

RICHARD T. McKEON, PhD, MPH
Senior Public Health Advisor, Center for Mental Health Services, SAMHSA, 988 and Behavioral Health Crisis Coordinating Office, Rockville, Maryland

ALEXANDER McCLANAHAN, MD, MHA
Resident Physician, Department of Psychiatry and Behavioral Sciences, Medical University of South Carolina, Charleston, South Carolina

COURTNEY L. McMICKENS, MD, MPH, MHS
Assistant Professor, Department of Psychiatry and Behavioral Sciences, Duke University, Durham, North Carolina; Associate Consultant, Lorio Forensics, Atlanta, Georgia

KENNETH MINKOFF, MD
Vice President and Chief Operating Officer, Psychiatrist, ZiaPartners, Inc, Catalina, Arizona

KERIS JÄN MYRICK, MBA, MS
Vice President of Partnerships, Inseparable, Washington, DC

STACY NONNEMACHER, PhD
Director of Cross System Strategies, NASDDS (National Association of State Directors of Developmental Disabilities Services), Alexandria, Vancouver

JOE PARKS, MD
Medical Director, National Council for Mental Wellbeing, Washington, DC

DEBRA A. PINALS, MD
Adjunct Clinical Professor, University of Michigan Medical School, Ann Arbor, Michigan; Director, Program in Psychiatry, Law, and Ethics, National Association of State Mental Health Program Directors

ANGELA PINHEIRO, MD, JD
Consultant, National Council for Mental Wellbeing, Okemos, Michigan

LEAH G. POPE, PhD
Associate Professor, Department of Psychiatry, Columbia University Vagelos College of Physicians and Surgeons, New York State Psychiatric Institute, New York, New York

JOHN S. ROZEL, MD, MSL
Professor of Psychiatry and Law, University of Pittsburgh, Medical Director, Resolve Crisis Services of UPMC Western Behavioral Health, Pittsburgh, Pennsylvania

MELISSA SCHOBER, MPM
Associate Professor, Innovations Institute, University of Connecticut School of Social Work, Hartford, Connecticut

BILLINA SHAW, MD, MPH
Senior Medical Advisor, Center for Mental Health Services, Substance Abuse and Mental Health Services Administration, Rockville, Maryland

SOSUNMOLU SHOYINKA, MD, MBA
Clinical Associate Professor of Psychiatry, University of Pennsylvania Perelman School of Medicine, Philadelphia, Pennsylvania; Centia Health PLLC, Media, Pennsylvania

LAYLA SOLIMAN, MD
Assistant Clinical Professor of Psychiatry, Atrium Health – Wake Forest Baptist School of Medicine, Charlotte, North Carolina

SARAH Y. VINSON, MD
Professor and Chair, Department of Psychiatry and Behavioral Sciences, Morehouse School of Medicine; Founder and Principal Consultant, Lorio Forensics; Adjunct Faculty, Department of Psychiatry and Behaivoral Scineces, Emory University, Lorio Forensics, Atlanta, Georgia

AMY C. WATSON, PhD
Professor, School of Social Work, Wayne State University, Detroit, Michigan

DEJUAN WHITE, MD
Assistant Professor, Department of Psychiatry and Behavioral Sciences, Emory University, Atlanta, Georgia

KAMILLE WILLIAMS, MD
Assistant Professor, Department of Psychiatry and Behavioral Sciences, Morehouse School of Medicine, Senior Associate, Lorio Forenscis, Atlanta, Georgia

MICHELLE ZABEL, MSS
Executive Director and Associate Extension Professor, Innovations Institute, University of Connecticut School of Social Work, Hartford, Connecticut

Contents

Crisis System Design & Accountability

Mental health crises among people who are marginalized merit special
consideration. These groups are both overserved and underserved by
mental health crisis systems: over-represented in acute treatment settings
by number while facing inequities in outcomes. The predisposing, precipitating, and perpetuating factors that contribute to crises, however, neither
begin nor end with the mental health system. Rather, these factors are
multisystemic. As an illustration of this concept, this article highlights select marginalized groups, those that have faced inequities in mental health
diagnosis and treatment due to race, medical complexity, age, and criminal justice system involvement.

This work expands on the National Council for Mental Wellbeing whitepaper Quality Measurement in Crisis Services. The authors present 2 approaches to measure development: The first maps flow through the
crisis continuum and defines metrics for each step of the process. The
second uses the mnemonic ACCESS TO HELP to define system values,
from the perspective of various stakeholders, with corresponding metrics.
The article also includes case examples and discusses how metrics can
align multiple components of a crisis system toward common goals, strategies for using metrics to drive quality improvement initiatives, and the
complexities of measuring and interpreting data.

The Crisis Continuum

This article reviews the historical trajectory of crisis hotlines in the United
States from their 1960's inception as 24/7 alternatives to traditional mental

health services to becoming "the front door" of the 988 Suicide and Crisis Lifeline in 2022. The Substance Abuse and Mental Health Services Administration's (SAMHSA's) 2001 effort to network, certify, and evaluate crisis hotlines laid the foundation for demonstrating the efficacy of crisis hotlines and their ability to reduce distress and suicidality in people accessing these services. SAMHSA-funded evaluations and the collective leadership of the National Suicide Prevention Lifeline network established evidence-based standards, policies, and practices.

Communities across the United States are working to improve community-based mental health crisis response, with 1 goal being to reduce criminal legal system involvement among individuals with mental illnesses, behavioral disorders, or mental health crises. Existing and recently developed models can generally be divided into non-law enforcement-based response models and law enforcement-based response models. Wide variation exists in terms of staffing, how response teams are called out or dispatched, hours of operation and immediacy of response, and approaches to crisis resolution.

Crisis facilities provide a safe and therapeutic alternative to emergency departments and jails for people experiencing behavioral health emergencies. Program design should center around customer needs which include individuals and families in crisis and key community stakeholders like first responders. Ideally, a crisis system should be organized into a broad continuum of services that ensures care is provided in the least restrictive setting, even for people with high acuity needs, and stakeholders should have a clear understanding of the capabilities of each component facility and the population it can safely serve. This paper provides a framework to help policymakers achieve this goal.

During the postcrisis period, many individuals struggle to transition to available care, often falling through the cracks. This article discusses effective postcrisis approaches that provide rapid access to transitional team-based care using critical time intervention strategies. It also highlights the development of state, county, and funder models for "care-traffic control" to ensure swift linkage to follow-up services, along with new funding models that support intensive community crisis stabilization during the postcrisis period. Emerging crisis systems can leverage these emerging services and approaches to facilitate successful transitions for individuals in need.

Clinical Practice in Crisis Services

Modern crisis centers need to be prepared for mass shootings, active assailant incidents, and related forms of targeted violence. While crisis engagement has traditionally been seen as a "right of boom" or post-incident responder, crisis leaders need to prepare their teams to identify people at risk for violence, use tools like Behavioral Threat Assessment and Management to reduce risk in those persons, and prepare their teams for potential incidents in their community. Evidence suggests that acute stressors are a common proximal risk factor for severe violence implying a potential synergy for using crisis services as a tool for prevention of violence.

Crisis response is growing across the United States with increasingly broad phone, text, and chat response systems that lead to triaging callers who may be in need of further outreach. This might include deploying a mobile crisis response team and/or referring a caller to a crisis stabilization unit. The information set forth earlier aims to help advance the field and individual practices to ensure that persons with intellectual and/or other developmental disorders receive equivalent care and treatment with information that helps focus on this population's unique features and needs.

People experiencing homelessness in crisis have unique structural vulnerabilities and social needs, most importantly lack of housing. Ideal crisis services for people experiencing homelessness must safeguard against criminalization and displacement during periods of crisis, prioritize equity, and provide housing interventions alongside mental health treatment at every stage in the crisis continuum. By outlining how to tailor crisis system financing and accountability, service component and capacity, and clinical best practices, the authors aim to provide hope and guidance for communities aiming to create an ideal crisis system for people experiencing homelessness.

The number of children and youth experiencing behavioral health crisis in the United States is substantially increasing. Currently, there are shortages to home-based and community-based services as well as psychiatric outpatient and inpatient pediatric care, leading to high emergency department utilization. This article introduces a proposed crisis continuum of care, highlights existing evidence, and provides opportunities for further research and advocacy.

Crisis Services

PSYCHIATRIC CLINICS OF NORTH AMERICA

SERIES OF RELATED INTEREST

Child and Adolescent Psychiatric Clinics of North America
https://www.childpsych.theclinics.com/

Neurologic Clinics
https://www.neurologic.theclinics.com/

Advances in Psychiatry and Behavioral Health
https://www.advancesinpsychiatryandbehavioralhealth.com/

THE CLINICS ARE AVAILABLE ONLINE!
Access your subscription at:
www.theclinics.com

Foreword

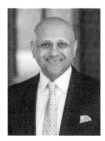

Harsh K. Trivedi, MD, MBA
Consulting Editor

The field of psychiatry is ever evolving, and the last few years have seen unprecedented change as we found ourselves in the midst of a global pandemic and then learned how to move forward in a post-COVID-19 world. From clinical and policy changes to new treatments and innovative research, our field continues to find new ways to adapt and care for those who are most vulnerable.

In 2008, I took over as consulting editor for *Child and Adolescent Psychiatric Clinics of North America* from Dr Andres Martin, and then as the inaugural editor of *Psychiatric Clinics of North America* in 2018. I am grateful for my time serving in those roles, as it was a true privilege to share my passion for the field and lend my knowledge and expertise as editor to the important topics that are covered in each and every issue. I hope I have contributed in some meaningful way to your knowledge base.

Throughout the years, we have covered critical issues, the latest trends, and the newest advancements and other topics important to psychiatry. From neuromodulation, to achieving mental health equity, sports psychiatry, workforce and diversity, adolescent cannabis use, and of course, how COVID-19 changed the profession, among many other topics.

The true value and benefit of a journal like this is the ability to go deep on topics that often don't receive the attention they deserve. By focusing on one topic per journal, with multiple articles and perspectives by leaders in those respective fields, there is the opportunity to drill down and truly get those unique perspectives.

I want to express my sincere thanks to all of the contributing authors and editors over the past number of years who have provided their expertise and knowledge. This knowledge helps educate other professionals in the field as we work to improve the health of our respective communities.

The value of any good journal is diversity of thought and perspectives that enrich and add depth to the field. In each of these series, I am proud to have left the *Psychiatric Clinics of North America* in a better spot and with more robust offerings than when I began as the editor. My hope is that this continues to be a series that is forward looking and thoughtful and that maintains its academic integrity well into the future.

Psychiatr Clin N Am 47 (2024) xi–xii
https://doi.org/10.1016/j.psc.2024.07.001
0193-953X/24/© 2024 Published by Elsevier Inc.

psych.theclinics.com

With this issue, I now hand over the proverbial baton to Dr Eric Storch, an experienced clinical psychologist with expertise in the assessment and treatment of children, adolescents, and adults with obsessive-compulsive and related disorders and anxiety disorders. He is a professor and the McIngvale Presidential Endowed Chair in the Department of Psychiatry and Behavioral Sciences at Baylor College of Medicine as well as serves as vice chair of psychology and head of psychology. As author of more than 800 articles and more than 20 books, he is a consummate educator and prolific writer. The series is in good hands, and I look forward to the forthcoming issues that he will contribute.

The future of our field is bright, and we can have significant impact across our communities. I eagerly await receiving upcoming issues, learning from our colleagues, and I wish the *Psychiatric Clinics of North America* continued success.

Harsh K. Trivedi, MD, MBA
Sheppard Pratt
6501 North Charles Street
Baltimore, MD 21204, USA

E-mail address:
htrivedi@sheppardpratt.org

Preface

Behavioral Health Crisis Services: From Policy to Practice

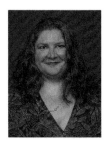 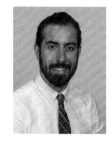

Margaret E. Balfour, MD, PhD   Matthew L. Goldman, MD, MS
Editors

There is a reckoning unfolding in psychiatric care across the United States: communities are confronting the limitations in access to treatment for mental health and substance use disorders and the inadequacy of a long-standing reliance on emergency medical services and criminal legal systems that struggle to care for people in crisis. As a result, there has been a surge in funding, system redesign, and program implementation that aims to expand the reach and impact of behavioral health crisis services. These specialized clinical services provide high-quality assessment, triage, interventions, and care coordination for people in the midst of acute psychiatric episodes related to both mental health and substance use, as well as intersecting physical comorbidities and social determinants of health.

This issue of *Psychiatric Clinics of North America* includes a range of important review articles that may serve as both a primer for clinicians who are less familiar with recent developments in behavioral health crisis services and a novel compilation of topics that have not previously been rigorously explored in such depth. The organization of this special issue mirrors a seminal report titled, "Roadmap to the Ideal Crisis System," authored by the Group for the Advancement of Psychiatry's Committee on Psychiatry and the Community and released by the National Council for Mental Wellbeing, which articulates three key areas that must be addressed to realize the vision of crisis services for all: (1) Crisis System Design and Accountability; (2) The Crisis Continuum; and (3) Clinical Practice in Crisis Services.

In the first section on crisis system design and accountability, authors Williams and colleagues make the case that advancement of mental health equity in crisis services requires a structurally informed approach that includes interpersonal, institutional, and societal level interventions and reforms that account for the impact of oppression and racism on mental health services. Hopper and colleagues then review the importance

Psychiatr Clin N Am 47 (2024) xiii–xv
https://doi.org/10.1016/j.psc.2024.04.021
0193-953X/24/© 2024 Published by Elsevier Inc.

of quality measurement and performance improvement in crisis systems, building on the prior article's emphasis that inequities must be measured and monitored for improvements as a way of holding systems accountable.

The next section includes four articles, each of which reviews the latest evidence for each component of the crisis continuum as described by the Substance Abuse and Mental Health Services Administration: someone to contact, someone to respond, and a safe place for help. Draper and McKeon, two of the most important leaders in advancing the growth of 988 and crisis services nationally, provide a historical perspective on the development of crisis hotlines in the United States. The topic of community-based mental health response, including mobile crisis and other models, is explored by Compton and colleagues, with a focus on implications for the workforce. Balfour and Carson provide a framework for organizing crisis facilities based on the acuity of individuals served and discuss strategies for designing crisis systems that meet the continuum of community and population needs. Finally, McClanahan and colleagues review the critical importance of, and approaches to, postcrisis follow-up for people who access crisis services and then need ongoing services and supports.

The final section on clinical best practices in crisis service settings begins with a review by Rozel and Soliman on approaches to preventing, surviving, and responding to active assailants, targeted violence, and mass violence. Anacker and colleagues review both diagnostic and treatment approaches for people with intellectual and/or other developmental disorders that must be addressed in crisis settings. The next article by Jackson and colleagues, addresses how specialized approaches that emphasize low-threshold access and engagement are needed for crisis services to best serve people experiencing homelessness. Finally, Foster and colleagues review how the crisis continuum must be adapted in to serve youth in crisis.

We hope the collection of articles in this issue of *Psychiatric Clinics of North America* will serve as a useful resource for clinicians, administrators, and policymakers as behavioral health crisis services continue to grow and evolve in the coming years.

DISCLOSURES

Dr M.E.Balfour has no conflicts of interest to disclose. Dr M.L. Goldman has no conflicts of interest to disclose. Dr M.L. Goldman receives research grant support from the National Institute of Mental Health (1R03MH130798).

Margaret E. Balfour, MD, PhD
Connections Health Solutions
2802 East District Street
Tucson, AZ 85714, USA

Department of Psychiatry
University of Arizona College of Medicine
Tucson, AZ, USA

Matthew L. Goldman, MD, MS
Department of Psychiatry and Behavioral Sciences
University of Washington
401 5th Avenue
Seattle, WA 98104, USA

Crisis Care Centers Initiative
King County Department of Community and Human Services
Seattle, WA, USA

E-mail addresses:
margie.balfour@connectionshs.org (M.E. Balfour)
mgoldma1@uw.edu (M.L. Goldman)

Crisis System Design & Accountability

Mental Health Crisis Responses and (In)Justice
Intrasystem and Intersystem Implications

Kamille Williams, MD[a],*, Alexis French, PhD[b],
Nicole Jackson, DSW, LCSW[c],
Courtney L. McMickens, MD, MPH, MHS[b,c], DeJuan White, MD[d],
Sarah Y. Vinson, MD[a,c,d]

KEYWORDS

- Crisis services • Medically complex • Youth
- Communities affected by mass incarceration • Carceral system-involved individuals

KEY POINTS

- The advancement of mental health equity requires a structurally informed approach, one that takes into account social, environmental, and cultural factors as well as the impact of oppression and racism on mental health symptom presentation and expression.
- Marginalization in the broader society is reflected in the experiences of those with mental health crises and who are seeking services.
- Addressing inequities in upstream structural and cultural drivers of poor population mental health is a critical component of mental health crisis reform discussion.
- Interpersonal, institutional, and societal level interventions and reform are needed to address the issues that contribute to mental health inequities.

INTRODUCTION

Mental health crises among people who are marginalized merit special consideration. These groups are both overserved and underserved by mental health crisis systems: over-represented in acute treatment settings by number while facing inequities in outcome.[1,2] The confluence of intersecting systems of oppression disproportionately

Funding support: The article was written without any funding.
[a] Department of Psychiatry and Behavioral Sciences, Morehouse School of Medicine, 720 Westview Drive Southwest, Atlanta, GA 30310, USA; [b] Department of Psychiatry and Behavioral Sciences, Duke University, 2608 Erwin Road, Durham, NC 27705, USA; [c] Lorio Forensics, 675 Seminole Avenue Northeast, Atlanta, GA 30307, USA; [d] Department of Psychiatry and Behavioral Sciences, Emory University, 12 Executive Park Drive Northeast, Atlanta, GA 30329, USA
* Corresponding author. Department of Psychiatry and Behavioral Sciences, Morehouse School of Medicine, 720 Westview Drive Southwest, Atlanta, GA, 30310.
E-mail address: Kwilliams@msm.edu

affects youth, Black and Latinx populations, as well as individuals with complex medical conditions and those incarcerated. Based on the published studies, these populations are typically the most impacted. These marginalized groups consistently confront adverse psychological and physical outcomes, characterized by limited reform. The predisposing, precipitating, and perpetuating factors that contribute to crises, however, neither begin nor end with the mental health system as these factors are multisystemic. The medical model, however, with its emphasis on the individual, is primed to underappreciate structural drivers, both within and beyond the health care system, of mental health crises and treatment experiences and their associated inequities.

Additionally, given the impact of cultural imperialism, which centers the experiences of dominant cultures, both the evaluation process and health care system delivery models often fail to account for the ways in which oppression and othering, or conceptualization of not belonging and differences that create marginalization and structural inequality, influence the expression and interpretations of mental health symptoms in marginalized populations.[3–5] Further, extant societal hierarchies may even be amplified in treatment settings, where medical culture is highly hierarchical, shaped by financial imperatives and fueled by a mental health workforce that is not representative of the larger population.[6] Inequity is also reflected in the medical literature, which is strikingly sparse for equity-centered crisis treatment articles.[6]

This article explores inequity in mental health crises and crisis care by highlighting intersystemic and intrasystemic considerations for several marginalized groups: those who have faced inequities in mental health diagnosis and treatment due to race, medical complexity, age, and criminal justice system influence and involvement. The various oppressive systems disproportionately affect these groups and the impact tends to be most pronounced and severe. Additionally, it offers prospective ideas for advancing equity in the burden, treatment, and understanding of mental health crises.

HIGHLIGHTED GROUPS
Minoritized Black and Latinx Populations

A fundamental driver of health inequities is structural racism, the totality of how societies support discrimination through mutually reinforcing systems and institutions that strengthen discriminatory beliefs, values, and inequitable distribution of power and resources.[7] One of the many consequences of structural racism is that it perpetuates educational, income, and wealth inequities, which in turn results in disparate access to adequate health insurance coverage and high-quality care.[8,9] Minoritized racial groups often experience more persistent and debilitating symptoms from their psychiatric conditions compared to white populations.[10,11] Further, Black and Latinx individuals are less likely to receive mental health treatment, and when they do, it is of less quantity and lower quality compared to White individuals.[12–16]

Minoritized racial groups face obstacles to accessing timely and culturally appropriate care as well as bias and discrimination in clinical practice.[13,17,18] Black and Latinx individuals are more likely to experience long wait times and lack of transportation when seeking medical care and have lower rates of insurance coverage than White individuals.[17,19] Given the inequities in community-based (as opposed to private) services on which these groups are more likely to depend due to wealth and income inequities, it follows that Black and Latinx individuals have higher rates of psychiatric emergency department visits compared to White individuals.[1,2] The inequities continue once these groups engage in crisis services. Black and Latinx patients presenting at the emergency departments for psychiatric reasons experience longer wait times and are more likely to receive chemical and physical restraint compared to White patients.[2,20–23]

Structural racism and individual bias not only interfere with receiving appropriate care but can also cause additional psychological distress and harm during a time of acute need. Research has demonstrated that providers' implicit biases can negatively impact patient–provider interactions as well as influence diagnostic and treatment decisions.[3,4] For instance, there exists a disproportionate diagnosis of psychotic disorders among Black and Latinx individuals in comparison to their White counterparts.[24] Misdiagnosis can result in inaccurate treatment, potentially intensifying symptoms and redirecting the focus of care from addressing the root cause to managing exacerbated symptoms. This, in turn, may contribute to the development of a complex medication regimen that inadvertently inflicts further harm.[3] Treating mental health concerns effectively in crisis care settings is challenging due to the need to quickly assess and triage patients to the appropriate level of care.[25,26] The fast-paced nature of mental health crisis evaluations, which are also high stakes and often performed by clinicians who have limited familiarity with the patient, renders these evaluations particularly vulnerable to the impact of racial bias on the interpretation of symptoms, the assessment of risk, the attribution of behaviors, and ultimately treatment.

Youth

Although often not included in discussions of underserved populations, population-based data and trends in access to care indicate that youth are a group that is inequitably served by the mental health care and crisis systems. In October 2021, the American Academy of Pediatrics, the American Academy of Child and Adolescent Psychiatry, and the Children's Hospital Association issued a joint statement declaring a national emergency in child and adolescent mental health.[27] The statement notes that in the decade leading up to the pandemic, youth rates of depression and anxiety were steadily increasing, as were rates of suicide and the use of emergency services for mental health concerns.[1,27] During and following COVID, suicide rates increased for adolescents and, in the wake of concurrent crises, death by overdose also continued to increase drastically among adolescents and young adults.[28] For youth, inequities in multiple societal systems that impact them are inextricably linked to psychological distress and acute mental health treatment needs.

The school system

Schools are a major source of youth mental health referrals to emergency departments—accounting for 25% of referrals.[29] School-based mental health services have been identified as ideal conduits for the promotion of positive social–emotional health, early identification of mental health symptoms, and provision of mental health care access throughout formative developmental stages.[30] Yet, there has been insufficient societal investment to realize the widespread and systematic implementation of these services. For some youth, the school setting is not only a place where there are missed opportunities regarding their mental health, but it is also one where they may be subjected to mental harm.

Youth experiences in schools have been associated with psychological distress due to interpersonal racism, biased educational expectations and disciplinary actions, and policies that entangle them in the criminal–legal system.[31,32] Further, the infrastructure of the public school system is built upon inequities, with persistent racial segregation and funding discrepancies.[33–35] These issues make it harder for school systems to provide the needed services to youth who face a disproportionate burden of adverse social determinants of health and are predictably at higher risk of mental health crisis.

The child welfare system

In the United States, it is estimated that nearly 400,000 youth are in foster care. Compared to the general population, these youth have higher rates of suicidality and suicidal behavior and are 3 to 4 times more likely to be diagnosed with mental illness.[36] Additionally, they are more likely to present with complex needs and psychosocial factors, such as those heavily influenced by the effects of disproportionate levels of poverty that affect mental health outcomes and access to care.[37,38] The child welfare system itself, which is vulnerable to underfunding and short staffing and also influenced by classism and racism, can introduce insecurity and further instability in key caregiver relationships. As a result, safety and security, bedrocks of mental well-being, are undermined for system-involved youth who are already at elevated risk of mental health issues due to the circumstances that led to child welfare engagement. Not surprisingly, involvement with child welfare has been associated with repeat visits for emergency psychiatric services.[39]

Multiply marginalized

Marginalized youth bear the brunt of the mental health crisis. Throughout the COVID-19 pandemic, the emergency departments were increasingly boarding children and adolescents with acute behavioral health needs. Youth identifying as Black, Latinx, or Spanish-speaking; lacking insurance coverage; showcasing trauma-related externalizing behaviors; and living with neurodevelopmental disorders were at higher risk of prolonged stays in the emergency department.[39–42] While sexual and gender minority youth are known to have higher rates of depression, anxiety, self-injurious behavior, and suicide attempts, little is known about the specific barriers to appropriate disposition following a visit for a mental health emergency,[43,44] representing a remarkable inequity in research and scholarship that negatively impacts the provision of services for this vulnerable group.

Medically Complex Populations

Individuals grappling with complex medical conditions encounter formidable obstacles when experiencing mental health crises. Remarkably, statistics suggest that nearly 1 in every 3 patients who are admitted to a general hospital inpatient unit contends with a psychiatric ailment.[45] Stringent medical clearance criteria, aimed at upholding the physical well-being of psychiatrically admitted patients, are required for admission into psychiatric hospitals. Typical exclusion parameters include anomalies in physical examinations, laboratory analyses, usage of assistive devices, and radiological assessments.[46] Individuals managing chronic illnesses demanding ongoing interventions, such as dialysis or dealing with irreversible co-occurring conditions such as neurologic and intellectual disability disorders, encounter challenges in accessing care within the acute care setting. This is often attributable to insufficient nursing and medical support in the inpatient psychiatric setting.[47] These phenomena underscore a widespread deficiency in the availability of acute care mental health beds for those across the medical spectrum. The foundation of exclusionary criteria in most psychiatric facilities revolves around institutional limitations, encompassing restricted access to emergent medical care, training limitations, and staff shortages for managing medically complex conditions.[48,49]

The prioritization of physical ailments or even idiosyncratic laboratory findings over mental ailments places medically complex psychiatric patients at a severe disadvantage in obtaining comprehensive mental health assessment and treatment. These patients, often confined to inpatient medical units, subsequently have their mental health care provided in a less psychologically therapeutic milieu and provided through the use of consultant liaison psychiatrists proffering recommendations for the overseeing hospitalist physician. This convergence of factors culminates in an extended duration of psychiatric care within medical facilities, yielding outcomes that include increased resource burden on the health care facilities and increased financial, emotional, and physical burden on patients.[49]

Multiply marginalized
Missed opportunities for upstream interventions are another important consideration for marginalized populations with medical comorbidities. A study conducted by Miller-Matero and colleagues underscored a disconcerting trend: racial and ethnic minorities who died by suicide exhibited a significantly elevated frequency of overall health visits on average compared to those who had not died by suicide.[50] Despite the presence of such compelling data, there has been insufficient study of suicide screening within outpatient medical clinical settings to inform interventions that are clearly evidence-based.[51] There is a notable void of clear directives for outpatient medical practitioners on how to effectively intervene for populations at high risk of crisis and suicidal outcomes even when concerns are identified. Older adults are another poorly served population as they endure prolonged stays in the emergency department, particularly when compounded by the presence of concurrent medical conditions.[52] Such prolonged sojourns within the emergency department have been intimately linked with escalated morbidity and mortality rates among the afflicted patients.

Populations Impacted by the Criminal–Legal System
Given the gaps in mental health crisis services, law enforcement officers (LEOs) are often first responders, despite having limited mental health training.[53,54] While fraught at baseline, in communities impacted by overpolicing and mass incarceration, the risks are even more pronounced. This is particularly relevant in the United States, which has the world's largest prison population, with approximately 358 adult state and federal prisoners per 100,000 citizens.[55] Mass incarceration disproportionately impacts marginalized populations and arises from a system deeply rooted in societal oppression.[56]

The concept of public safety has been distorted by policies that initiated and continue to endorse proactive policing practices, aggressive prosecution, and harsh sentencing terms—framed as the need to protect the community against dangerous predators, unsafe city streets, and high rates of crime.[57] Promoting such images and language permits targeting vulnerable populations and their labeling as societal menaces. Consequently, those in need of mental health crisis services, who are also members of affected communities, are primed to have negative associations with LEOs—and vice versa.

Law enforcement officers as first responders and safety professionals
LEO encounters pose unique risks to those in mental health crisis. During police interactions, individuals with a mental health condition are 16 times more likely to die compared to those without a mental health condition,[58,59] and Black individuals with a mental health condition are 2.8 times more likely to die than White individuals.[60,61] Furthermore, the effects of discriminatory policing and police brutality have profound effects on one's mental health and morbidity—feeding stressors that may contribute to crisis states.[58–63] With the launch of 988 and other crisis programs, it will be critical

to evaluate both the implementation and outcomes by responder type, LEO versus mental health professional versus co-responder models and to stratify data in a manner that allows for detection of inequities along categories such as race, class, and disability.[6] Achieving this requires the direct engagement of communities in crisis system design guided by a globally adopted equity framework which measures progress and promotes organizational accountability across systems.

Formerly incarcerated individuals

Those returning to society after imprisonment are another group at high risk for unaddressed mental health concerns increasing vulnerability to mental health crises. Privatizing prisons has further complicated the already fraught relationship between incarceration and health, as these for-profit companies' bottom lines depend on increased incarceration rates and minimal spending on staffing and programming.[64] These companies have no financial incentive to mitigate the costs of failed societal re-entry for returning citizens. Limited access to educational, vocational, and mental health services perpetuates structural disadvantages and dims the prospect of successful societal re-entry. Effectively, when released, those now classified as "ex-offenders" frequently return to their communities with limited job skills and occupational prospects, placing them at risk for significant adverse social determinants of mental health such as poverty and homelessness. These are ingredients for community, family, and individual destabilization, and create circumstances rife for mental health crises.

The relationship between the carceral system and acute mental health care needs implicates issues beyond individual choice and biological risk factors. However, narratives of those who are deemed "criminals and delinquents" can undermine much needed exploration and reform. The structural lens needed to fully understand health inequities can also be applied to those at disproportionate risk of contact with the legal system. Perhaps it is necessary to question the stance that criminal behavior is an individual moral choice rather than a response to structural conditions, economic inequality, or discriminatory injustices.[58]

DISCUSSION

A social justice lens, one that recognizes that the social determinants of mental health are in fact shaped by the unfair and inequitable distribution of resources and opportunity, supports a structurally informed approach to mental health crisis evaluation and systems change. An understanding of where the mental health crisis system falls short, and how to improve outcomes, includes awareness of the unique barriers to more upstream and community-based interventions for marginalized populations while also accounting for relevant societal systems' differential treatment of them.

This article highlights intersystemic and intrasystemic contributors to inequitable, discriminatory, and biased mental health crisis care. Gaps in literature and perpetuation of societal hierarchies within the health care system contribute to inaccurate diagnoses, inappropriate treatment, and even at times traumatic experiences due to aggressive mental health interventions or excessive use of force by LEOs. Deliberate consideration of marginalized populations should be at the forefront of designing systems and delivering treatments for mental health crises prevention and response at the local, state, and national levels. A vital step involves redesigning economic, social, and political structures with a central goal of dismantling racism and other forms of discrimination within the mental health system.

The declaration of a national emergency in child and adolescent mental health must be followed by action, serving as a clarion call for meaningful financial investment in systems that allow for early identification of mental health symptoms and connection to mental health care. Additionally, it is critical that school systems re-examine and correct for harsh disciplinary practices that foster psychological distress and pose the threat of initiation in the school-to-prison pipeline. Further, given the clear vulnerability of youth in the child welfare system and those from minoritized groups, be it by race, sexual orientation, and or gender identity, research, evaluation, and interventions specifically for these groups is sorely needed.

For the patient who has both medically and psychiatrically complex conditions, the prioritization of physical health over mental health results in suboptimal care at the time of mental health crises. Greater integration of medical and mental health services, in primary care, outpatient mental health, and acute treatment settings, would support treatment improvements in this group. There is also need for more studies of training in the primary care setting for mental health crisis prevention. Numerous publications discuss United States Preventive Services Task Force (USPSTF) recommendations for mental health screening and intervention in the primary care setting.[65] Despite this wealth of information, the USPTF lacks enough evidence to support recommendations to screen and/or intervene suicide risk or address other mental health crises in the primary care setting.[66] The uncertainty surrounding this issue raises questions about the comfort level of primary care physicians in providing such interventions, possibly stemming from training limitations. Studies reveal that 45% of individuals who died by suicide had consulted with their primary care physician within 30 days of the attempt.[67] Therefore, there exists a substantial opportunity to enhance primary care physicians' ability to identify and address suicide and mental health concerns.

Far from therapeutic, interactions with LEOs can be not only distressing but also fatal, particularly for marginalized individuals with mental illness. With the increased attention to mental health crisis response and the ongoing rollout of 988, there is a valuable opportunity to diminish the involvement of LEOs in mental health crisis response and for the mental health care systems to take its rightful place in the lead. Finally, given returning citizens' predictably high risk of experiencing adverse social determinants of health, special attention should be given to outreach, upstream intervention, and mental health treatment accessibility for them, a group that makes up a substantial portion of the US society given its extraordinary rates of incarceration.

SUMMARY

Addressing the demand for and the inequities in crisis mental health simply cannot begin and end with 911, 988, emergency departments, or even the outpatient mental health care system. Population-responsive community-based programs as well as addressing upstream predictive, precipitating, and perpetuating factors at a population level are key.[53] As the drivers of mental health crises are multisystemic, an effective response, one that includes both prevention and intervention, must transcend siloed systems and take great care in documenting—and addressing—inequities and discrimination in all its forms.

CLINICS CARE POINTS

- Mental health crisis care system design and clinical assessment should be structurally informed, taking into account social and environmental factors as well as the impact of marginalization on symptom presentation and expression.

- Clinicians must consider how both their own biases and the culture of medicine/mental health care may adversely influence the assessment and treatment process for marginalized groups.
- Child welfare, school, and mental health systems and their professionals should be aware of and appropriately funded to account for the vulnerability of youth, especially those who face multiple forms of marginalization.
- Individuals with medically complex conditions in mental health crises have hardships receiving quality care, and an interdisciplinary orientation and leadership in better integration of services is required to care for them more optimally.
- The unnecessary involvement of LEOs poses both psychological and physical risk to those in mental health crises and should be minimized and ideally eliminated.
- The development of standardized training in integrated care may help medical and mental health providers and staff improve the quality of care for those with comorbid mental and medical conditions.
- The gaps in research related to marginalized populations and mental health crises and treatment must be narrowed through intentional engagement with and support of researcher collaborators with connection, commitment, and expertise in providing care to marginalized communities.

DISCLOSURE

Dr S.Y. Vinson is the Founder and Principal Consultant of Lorio Forensics. Dr C.L. McMickens is a contract associate consultant of Lorio Forensics.

REFERENCES

1. Abrams AH, Badolato GM, Boyle MD, et al. Racial and ethnic disparities in pediatric mental health-related emergency department visits. Pediatr Emerg Care 2022;38(1):e214–8.
2. Peters ZJ, Santo L, Davis D, et al. Emergency Department visits related to mental health disorders among adults, by race and hispanic ethnicity: United States, 2018-2020. Natl Health Stat Report 2023;181:1–9.
3. Hall WJ, Chapman MV, Lee KM, et al. Implicit racial/ethnic bias among health care professionals and its influence on health care outcomes: a systematic review. Am J Publ Health 2015;105(12):e60–76.
4. FitzGerald C, Hurst S. Implicit bias in healthcare professionals: a systematic review. BMC Med Ethics 2017;18:19.
5. Akbulut N, Razum O. Why othering should be considered in research on health inequalities: Theoretical Perspectives and Research needs. SSM - Population Health 2022;20:101286.
6. Goldman ML, Vinson SY. Centering equity in mental health crisis services. World Psychiatr 2022;21(2):243–4.
7. Bailey ZD, Krieger N, Agénor M, et al. Structural racism and health inequities in the USA: evidence and interventions. Lancet 2017;389(10077):1453–63.
8. Yearby R. Structural racism and health disparities: reconfiguring the social determinants of health framework to include the root cause. J Law Med Ethics 2020; 48(3):518–26.
9. Yearby R, Clark B, Figueroa JF. Structural racism in Historical And Modern US Health Care Policy. Health Aff 2022;41(2):187–94.
10. Bailey RK, Mokonogho J, Kumar A. Racial and ethnic differences in depression: current perspectives. Neuropsychiatric Dis Treat 2019;15:603–9.

11. Williams DR, González HM, Neighbors H, et al. Prevalence and distribution of major depressive disorder in African Americans, Caribbean blacks, and non-Hispanic whites: results from the National Survey of American Life. Arch Gen Psychiatr 2007;64:305–15.
12. 2015 National healthcare quality and disparities report: chartbook on health care for blacks. Rockville (MD): Agency for Healthcare Research and Quality (US); 2016. Available at: https://www.ahrq.gov/sites/default/files/wysiwyg/research/findings/nhqrdr/chartbooks/qdr2015-chartbook-blacks.pdf. [Accessed 8 August 2023].
13. McGuire TG, Miranda J. New evidence regarding racial and ethnic disparities in mental health: policy implications. Health Aff 2008;27(2):393–403.
14. Alegria M, Vallas M, Pumariega AJ. Racial and ethnic disparities in pediatric mental health. Child Adolesc Psychiatr Clin N Am 2010;19(4):759–74.
15. Lasser KE, Himmelstein DU, Woolhandler SJ, et al. Do minorities in the United States receive fewer mental health services than whites? Int J Health Serv 2002; 32(3):567–78.
16. Cook BL, Zuvekas SH, Carson N, et al. Assessing racial/ethnic disparities in treatment across episodes of mental health care. Health Serv Res 2014;49(1):206–29.
17. Caraballo C, Ndumele CD, Roy B, et al. Trends in racial and ethnic disparities in barriers to timely medical care among adults in the US, 1999 to 2018. JAMA Health Forum 2022;3(10):e223856.
18. Chapman EN, Kaatz A, Carnes M. Physicians and implicit bias: how doctors may unwittingly perpetuate health care disparities. J Gen Intern Med 2013;28(11): 1504–10.
19. US Census. Health Insurance Coverage in the United States. 2015. Available at: https://www.census.gov/content/dam/Census/library/publications/2016/demo/p60-257.pdf. [Accessed 8 August 2023].
20. Goldfarb SS, Graves K, Geletko K, et al. Racial and Ethnic Differences in Emergency Department Wait Times for Patients with Substance Use Disorder. J Emerg Med 2023;64(4):481–7.
21. Khatri UG, Delgado MK, South E, et al. Racial disparities in the management of emergency department patients presenting with psychiatric disorders. Ann Epidemiol 2022;69:9–16.
22. Smith CM, Turner NA, Thielman NM, et al. Association of black race with physical and chemical restraint use among patients undergoing emergency psychiatric evaluation. Psychiatr Serv 2022;73(7):730–6.
23. Carreras Tartak JA, Brisbon N, Wilkie S, et al. Racial and ethnic disparities in emergency department restraint use: A multicenter retrospective analysis. Acad Emerg Med 2021;28(9):957–65.
24. Schwartz RC, Blankenship DM. Racial disparities in psychotic disorder diagnosis: A review of empirical literature. World J Psychiatr 2014;4(4):133–40.
25. Slade EP, Dixon LB, Semmel S. Trends in the duration of emergency department visits, 2001–2006. Psychiatr Serv 2010;61:878–84.
26. Zun LS. Pitfalls in the care of the psychiatric patient in the emergency department. J Emerg Med 2012;43:829–35.
27. A declaration from the American Academy of Pediatrics. American Academy of Child and Adolescent Psychiatry and Children's Hospital Association. 2021. Available at: https://www.aap.org/en/advocacy/child-and-adolescent-healthy-mental-development/aap-aacap-cha-declaration-of-a-national-emergency-in-child-and-adolescent-mental-health/.

28. Panchal NR. Robin; Cox, Cynthia. Recent trends in mental health and substance use concerns among adolescents. *Issue Brief*. KFF; 2022. Available at: https://www.kff.org/coronavirus-covid-19/issue-brief/recent-trends-in-mental-health-and-substance-use-concerns-among-adolescents/. [Accessed 20 March 2023].

29. Oblath R, Oh A, Herrera CN, et al. Psychiatric emergencies among urban youth during COVID-19: Volume and acuity in a multi-channel program for the publicly insured. J Psychiatr Res 2023;160:71–7.

30. Flaherty LT, Weist MD, Warner BS. School-based mental health services in the united states: History, current models and needs. journal article. Community Ment Health J 1996;32(4):341–52.

31. Fadus MC, Valadez EA, Bryant BE, et al. Racial disparities in elementary school disciplinary actions: findings from the ABCD study. J Am Acad Child Adolesc Psychiatr 2021;60(8):998–1009.

32. Crutchfield J, Phillippo KL, Frey A. Structural racism in schools: a view through the lens of the National School Social work practice model. article. Child Sch 2020;42(3):187–93.

33. Allegretto S, García E, Weiss E. Public education funding in the U.S. needs an overhaul: How a larger federal role would boost equity and shield children from disinvestment during downturns. 2022. epi.org/233143.

34. McGrew W. US school segregation in the 21st century. Causes, consequences, and solutions. Washington DC: Washington Center for Equitable Growth; 2019.

35. Zeimer S. Exclusionary Zoning, School Segregation, and Housing Segregation: An Investigation into a Modern Desegregation Case and Solutions to Housing Segregation Note. Hastings Consititut Law Q 2020;48(1):205–30.

36. Engler AD, Sarpong KO, Van Horne BS, et al. A systematic review of mental health disorders of children in foster care. Trauma Violence Abuse 2020;23(1):255–64.

37. Leslie LK, Landsverk J, Ezzet-Lofstrom R, et al. Children in foster care: factors influencing outpatient mental health service use. Child Abuse Negl 2000;24(4):465–76.

38. Eckenrode J, Smith EG, McCarthy ME, et al. Income inequality and child maltreatment in the United States. Pediatrics (Evanston) 2014;133(3):454–61.

39. Marr M, Horwitz S, Gerson R, et al. Friendly faces: characteristics of children and adolescents with repeat visits to a specialized child psychiatric emergency program. friendly faces: characteristics of children and adolescents with repeat visits to a specialized child psychiatric emergency program. Pediatr Emerg Care 2021;37(1):4–10.

40. Smith JL, De Nadai AS, Petrila J, et al. Factors associated with length of stay in emergency departments for pediatric patients with psychiatric problems. Pediatr Emerg Care 2019;35(10):716–21.

41. Brathwaite D, Strain A, Waller AE, et al. The effect of increased emergency department demand on throughput times and disposition status for pediatric psychiatric patients. Am J Emerg Med 2023;64:174–83.

42. McMickens CL, Maslow G, Keeshin B. Child Welfare Interventions and system transformation to improve the lives of children and families who experience trauma. J Am Acad Child Adolesc Psychiatr 2022;61(10, Supplement):S60.

43. Hoffmann JA, Alegría M, Alvarez K, et al. Disparities in pediatric mental and behavioral health conditions. Pediatrics 2022;150(4).

44. McEnany FB, Ojugbele O, Doherty JR, et al. Pediatric mental health boarding. Pediatrics 2020;146(4).

45. Van Niekerk M, Walker J, Hobbs H, et al. The prevalence of psychiatric disorders in general hospital inpatients: a systematic umbrella review. J Acad Consult Liaison Psychiatry 2022;63(6):567–78.
46. Moukaddam N, Udoetuk S, Tucci V, et al. Exclusionary criteria for inpatient hospitalization: Quality safeguards or unnecessary roadblocks? Psychiatr Ann 2018;48(1):51–7.
47. Tucci V, Liu J, Matorin A, et al. Like the eye of the tiger: inpatient psychiatric facility exclusionary criteria and its "knockout" of the emergency psychiatric patient. J Emerg Trauma Shock 2017;10(4):189–93.
48. Certa K. Medically and psychiatrically complicated patients. Psychiatr Times 2017. Available at: https://www.psychiatrictimes.com/view/medically-and-psychiatrically-complicated-patients. [Accessed 23 January 2024].
49. Lyketsos CG, Dunn G, Kaminsky MJ, et al. Medical comorbidity in psychiatric inpatients: relation to clinical outcomes and hospital length of stay. Psychosomatics 2002;43(1):24–30.
50. Miller-Matero LR, Yeh H-H, Maffett A, et al. Racial-ethnic differences in receipt of past-year health care services among suicide decedents: A case-control study. Psychiatr Serv 2023. https://doi.org/10.1176/appi.ps.20220578.
51. O'Connor E, Gaynes B, Burda BU, et al. Screening for suicide risk in primary care: a systematic evidence Review for the U.S. Preventive services Task force. Rockville (MD): Agency for Healthcare Research and Quality (US); 2013.
52. Rhodes SM, Patanwala AE, Cremer JK, et al. Predictors of prolonged length of stay and adverse events among older adults with behavioral health-related emergency department visits: a systematic medical record review. J Emerg Med 2016; 50(1):143–52.
53. Pinals DA, Edwards ML. Law enforcement and crisis services: Past Lessons for New Partnerships and the Future of 988. Technical assistance collaborative Paper No. 4. Alexandria, VA: National Association of State Mental Health Program Directors; 2021.
54. Tartaro C, Bonnan-White J, Mastrangelo M, et al. Police Officers attitudes toward mental health and crisis intervention: understanding preparedness to respond to community members in crisis. J Police Crim Psychol 2021;36:579–91.
55. Carson EA. Prisoners in 2020–Statistical tables. NCJ 2021;302776:1–50.
56. Brinkley-Rubinstein L, Cloud DH. Mass incarceration as a social-structural driver of health inequities: a supplement to *AJPH*. Am J Publ Health 2020;110(S1): S14–5.
57. Garland D. The current crisis of American Criminal Justice: A structural analysis. Annual Review of Criminology 2023;6(1):43–63.
58. Fuller DA, Lamb R, Biasotti M, et al. Overlooked in the undercounted: the role of mental illness in fatal law enforcement encounters. Treatment Advocacy Center 2015. Available at: http://www.treatmentadvocacycenter.org/storage/documents/overlooked-in-the-undercounted.pdf. [Accessed 8 August 2023].
59. Lane-McKinley K, Tsungmey T, Roberts LW. The Deborah Danner Story: Officer-Involved Deaths of People Living with Mental Illness. Acad Psychiatr 2018;42(4): 443–50.
60. Shadravan SM, Edwards ML, Vinson SY. Dying at the intersections: police-involved killings of black people with mental illness. Psychiatr Serv 2021;72(6): 623–5.
61. DeGue S, Fowler KA, Calkins C. Deaths due to use of lethal force by law enforcement: findings from the National Violent Death Reporting System, 17 US states, 2009-2012. Am J Prev Med 2016;51(suppl 3):S173–87.

62. Boyd RW. Police violence and the built harm of structural racism. Lancet 2018; 392(10144):258–9.
63. DeVylder J, Fedina L, Link B. Impact of police violence on mental health: a theoretical framework. Am J Publ Health 2020;110(11):1704–10.
64. Kim D-Y. Prison privatization: an empirical literature review and path forward. Int Crim Justice Rev 2019;32(1):24–47.
65. Barry MJ, Nicholson WK, Silverstein M, et al. Screening for depression and suicide risk in adults. JAMA 2023;329(23):2057.
66. Horowitz LM, Bridge JA, Tipton MV, et al. Implementing suicide risk screening in a pediatric primary care setting: From research to practice. Acad Pediatr 2022; 22(2):217–26.
67. Mangione CM, Barry MJ, Nicholson WK, et al. Screening for depression and suicide risk in children and adolescents. JAMA 2022;328(15):1534.

Multidimensional Approaches to Quality Measurement and Performance Improvement in the Ideal Crisis System

Ken Hopper, MD, MBA[a], Angela Pinheiro, MD, JD[b],
Sosunmolu Shoyinka, MD, MBA[c,d], Joe Parks, MD[e],
Kenneth Minkoff, MD[f], Billina Shaw, MD, MPH[g],
Matthew L. Goldman, MD, MS[h], Margaret E. Balfour, MD, PhD[i,j,*]

KEYWORDS

- Quality improvement • Mental health services • Crisis intervention
- Emergency psychiatric services • Healthcare quality indicators • Hotlines

KEY POINTS

- The crisis field is evolving rapidly, and quality metrics are needed to demonstrate value and success, inform quality improvement efforts, and maintain a focus on the needs of service users.
- Crisis systems exist within a larger healthcare ecosystem with many stakeholders including patients, families, crisis providers, contiguous health services, law enforcement, payers, social service organizations, and others.
- Systems engineering approaches map of how individuals move through the crisis system and create metrics focused on each of the major steps or "zones" – community, triage/ intake, crisis intervention, discharge planning and execution, and post-discharge services.

Continued

[a] Alice L. Walton School of Medicine, 1110 Northeast Fillmore Street, Bentonville, AR 72712, USA; [b] National Council for Mental Wellbeing, 3676 Fairhills Drive, Okemos, MI 48864, USA; [c] Centia Health PLLC, 36 East Front Street, Media, PA 19063, USA; [d] University of Pennsylvania Perelman School of Medicine, Philadelphia, PA, USA; [e] National Council for Mental Wellbeing, 1400 K Street Northwest Suite 400, Washington, DC 20005, USA; [f] Zia Partners, Inc, 15270 North Oracle Road, Suite 124-308, Catalina, AZ 85739, USA; [g] Center for Mental Health Services, Substance Abuse and Mental Health Services Administration, 5600 Fishers Lane, Rockville, MD 20857, USA; [h] Department of Psychiatry and Behavioral Sciences, University of Washington, King County Department of Community and Human Resources, 401 5th Avenue, Seattle, WA 98104, USA; [i] Connections Health Solutions, 2802 East District Street, Tucson, AZ 85714, USA; [j] Deparment of Psychiatry, University of Arizona College of Medicine, Tucson, AZ, USA
* Corresponding author.
E-mail address: margie.balfour@connectionshs.org

Psychiatr Clin N Am 47 (2024) 457–472
https://doi.org/10.1016/j.psc.2024.04.002   **psych.theclinics.com**

Continued

- Person-centered approaches translate system values into metrics. The authors use the mnemonic ACCESS TO HELP to describe a core set of values for crisis systems. Each value is defined in non-technical customer-focused language and mapped to example metrics.
- Measuring systemwide performance aligns the multiple processes and components of the system toward common goals. This provides a foundation for systems to identify areas needing improvement and work together to improve performance.

INTRODUCTION

Crisis Services are necessary to help those with unexpected emergencies and circumstances. As with all emergency management situations in healthcare, each crisis event provides an opportunity to explore contributors to the crisis and to deploy optimally efficient methods to resolve it. Crisis systems aim to provide rapid access to care for individuals experiencing mental health challenges, and to alleviate distress as quickly, safely, and effectively as possible. Mental health crisis systems across the country are developing rapidly as local, state, and national resources have been earmarked to address issues such as emergency department (ED) boarding, unnecessary law enforcement involvement in responses to non-criminal health care crises, and inadequate and inequitable access to mental health care services.

This writing complements and expands the logic outlined in *Quality Measurement in Crisis Services*, a whitepaper released by The National Council for Mental Wellbeing in early 2023.[1] Our approach recognizes that communities across the United States are in different stages of development in building and expanding crisis services and that the field is rapidly evolving. Rather than generate a prescriptive list of metrics, the authors aim to provide a guide to help leaders and stakeholders think about and select metrics relevant to their organizations and communities. The authors present 2 approaches to measure development: The first is process-based and involves mapping flow through the various parts of the crisis continuum then selecting metrics that reflect how well each step was performed. The second is person-centered and uses the mnemonic ACCESS TO HELP to define system values, from the perspective of the customer, with corresponding metrics. The authors also discuss how metrics can align the multiple components of a crisis system toward common goals, strategies for using metrics to drive continuous quality improvement (CQI) initiatives, and the complexities of measuring and interpreting data.

A BALANCED PERSPECTIVE

As crisis systems evolve across the country, organizations and other stakeholders continue to re-think the meaning of "quality" in this context. This requires systems to define desired outcomes and value from the perspective of multiple stakeholders. Tension can arise when a positive outcome for one stakeholder group may result in negative outcomes for others. For example, cost savings for payers may come at the cost of diminished outcomes for service users because of inadequate funding for needed services. For this reason, a balanced scorecard is recommended. This term refers to a transparent process where outcomes from multiple perspectives are weighed and evaluated to provide a more holistic view of the overall outcomes and quality of care. The Institute of Healthcare Improvement's Quintuple Aim Framework offers an

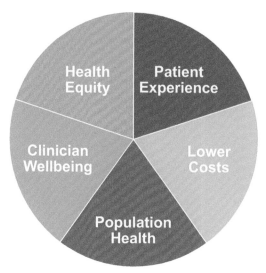

Fig. 1. The quintuple aim–a multidimensional quality framework.

excellent example of a balanced scorecard approach, defining healthcare quality across 5 dimensions comprised of patient experience, cost of care, population health, experience of clinicians, and health equity.[2] (**Fig. 1**).

Crisis systems in particular span many silos, and the stakeholders are many and varied, including.

- Individual patients
- Involved families
- Crisis service providers
- First responders (Law enforcement, emergency medical services, and so forth.)
- Contiguous healthcare services (EDs, hospitals, community behavioral health providers, and primary care providers)
- Social service organizations (homeless services, child welfare agencies, and so forth.)
- Public safety and criminal justice systems
- Schools
- Funders of care
- State and local governments
- Communities
- Society-at-large

QUALITY METRICS WITHIN THE TOTAL SYSTEM OF HEALTHCARE

All systems are essentially an aggregation of linked processes working in concert to achieve and consistently replicate specific and intended outcomes. However, these processes are prone to error (human and otherwise), and few are as complex as the web of services that make up a mental health crisis care continuum.

Clinical intervention systems that alleviate distress and drive clinical outcomes operate within the context of larger systems of care. These interlocking systems are increasingly referred to as *ecosystems*.[3] The term "ecosystem" refers to a network

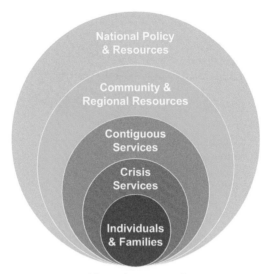

Fig. 2. The healthcare ecosystem–crisis service perspective.

of interfacing, mutually dependent parts of a system that must work together to achieve target outcomes.

Healthcare systems of care (termed ecosystems in this article) comprise organizations that provide direct clinical services, as well as agencies tasked with oversight, funding, care and quality management, community safety, and psychosocial support. It also includes individuals that use these services, their families, and other stakeholders (**Fig. 2**).

For ecosystems to be maximally effective, high levels of cooperation, trust, collaboration, and transparency must exist. Given the complexities inherent in healthcare ecosystems and the high-stakes nature of the work, workflow/process design, or "systems engineering" is essential to create workflows and pathways that increase efficiency, reduce risk, and optimize outcomes.

Used in this context, the term "engineering" refers to an intentional, proactive, and systematic process of creating (designing) workflows that drive desired outcomes. The standardized preflight checklist process within the aviation industry is an example of process engineering. These workflows were created to reduce avoidable mechanical and human error and to maximize safety for travelers.

The need for systems engineering or process design is increasingly recognized within healthcare because of the ever-evolving complexity of these environments and a need to optimize efficiency, productivity, and outcomes. Health Systems Science is now considered a fundamental discipline within the healthcare industry and health education. As in other industries, healthcare systems must strive to create a culture that embraces continuous quality improvement with thoughtful use of metrics that track performance in critical operational areas and that monitor key outcomes. For a field like crisis care, which in many communities is still in early stages of development, quality metrics not only monitor performance of existing services and processes but also identify care gaps that can help community leaders prioritize investment in additional infrastructure, services, or training.

FRAMEWORKS AND PERSPECTIVES IN CRISIS METRICS
Types of Measures

When selecting metrics, it is important to understand the various types of measures and when their application is most effective to support quality management and performance improvement efforts. Avedis Donabedian–an early pioneer of quality measurement in healthcare–developed the commonly-used framework for classifying measures into 3 types: structure, process, and outcome.[4]

- *Structure metrics* ask "What do you HAVE?" and include measures of the care environment and infrastructure such as staffing, space, software, and technology. Examples: Is there 24/7 coverage by a psychiatrist? Is there an electronic bed registry?
- *Process metrics* ask "What did you DO?" and indicate whether workflows are performing as designed, so that problems can be quicky detected and improved using process engineering methods. Examples: Door to assessment time, time from dispatch to arrival time for mobile crisis teams, percent of patients screened for domestic violence and so forth
- *Outcome metrics* ask "Did it WORK?" and refer to well-chosen, critical-to-success service result measures. Examples:
  - Clinical: Did both objective and subjective signs of "the clinical condition" improve? Were there improvements in functioning and quality of life?
  - Satisfaction: Did "stakeholder" find crisis services to be "positive attribute"?
  - Efficiency: Were there fewer "steps, transitions, and hospitalizations" because of the service?

In general, outcome measures are considered the most desirable but are often also the hardest to measure. More recently there has been increased attention on measuring outcomes that are meaningful to the patient and developing Patient Reported Outcome Measures [5] that capture quality of life, functional status, and patient experience. However, structure and process metrics can also be quite useful, especially for crisis systems that are still growing and developing.

Hermann and Palmer describe additional considerations to guide the selection of useful metrics.[6] They outline a simple and pragmatic set of criteria that metrics be meaningful, feasible, and actionable.

- *Meaningful:* Does the measure reflect a process that is clinically important? Is there evidence supporting the measure? Compared with other fields, there is a less robust evidence base for behavioral health measures, so we must often rely on face validity or adapt measures for which there is evidence in other settings, such as call centers and EDs.
- *Feasible:* Is it possible to collect the data needed for the measure? If so, can this be done accurately, quickly, and easily, with a minimum of manual audits? Data must be produced within a short timeframe to be actionable.
- *Actionable*: Do the measures provide direction for future improvement activities? Are there established benchmarks toward which to strive? Are the factors leading to suboptimal performance within the span of control of the system to address?

Traditionally, healthcare measures capture data from events that have already occurred. Systems engineering can incorporate real-time performance monitoring that identifies potential problems result of which they can be addressed as they occur ("quality at the source"). The Universal Protocol or "time out" performed in hospital settings to reduce medical errors is a good example of an engineered protocol.

Measurement in the context of engineered pathways focuses on fidelity to pathway logic (process/workflows) and when there should be exceptions or escalation to a higher level of care or leadership involvement. Although this approach has the potential to prevent harm and adverse outcomes before they reach individual patients and reduce the need for more time-consuming and costly methods of quality oversight, the healthcare industry has been late in adopting these principles compared with other industries like aviation and manufacturing.[7,8]

Finally, it is important to have clearly defined and standardized definitions for each metric. A "measure specification" is a set of instructions for how to build and calculate a measure.[9] Each measure specification includes an "operational definition" that describes how to calculate the measure by precisely defining the numerator, denominator, start and end points of time measures, included and excluded populations, and measure logic. Specifications also include details about the target population, data sources, the rationale and evidence for using the measure, and considerations for interpreting the metrics. Individual organizations then use these definitions to develop processes to extract data from their electronic health record (EHR), claims database, and so forth,. and calculate the measure.

Standardized measure specifications ensure that everyone is measuring the same way and are critical for making valid comparisons and establishing national or community-wide performance benchmarks. For this reason, national organizations may develop or endorse measures to create industry standards. The Partnership for Quality Measurement maintains a searchable database of measure specifications endorsed by the Center for Medicare and Medicaid Services (CMS).[10] The National Center for Quality Assurance (NCQA) maintains the Healthcare Effectiveness Data and Information Set (HEDIS) measures that are used by health plans.[11] Adopting (or closely adapting) existing and endorsed measures can help crisis systems develop quality measures that facilitate comparisons or benchmarking and fit into the larger healthcare ecosystem.

A Process-Based Framework for Crisis Metrics

The process-workflow diagram portrayed in **Fig. 3** provides a high-level map of how individuals move through the crisis system with the major steps divided into "zones" – community, triage or intake, crisis intervention, discharge planning and execution, and post-discharge services. At each zone, a consideration of the relevant inputs, outputs, gaps, and best-practices provides a starting place for developing metrics. The authors discuss and provide examples for each zone as follows.

Community

Is the community aware of crisis services, and can they use the services easily? A recent Pew survey[12] illustrates the importance of addressing these questions. Nine months after the launch of 988, 18% reported they had heard of 988, but of that group, only 26% reported they didn't know or weren't sure when someone should contact it. The survey also identified barriers to using 988, which includes concerns about police involvement, involuntary hospitalization, privacy, ability to pay, and whether the call-takers would be able to address their need. This data provide important information about where to target improvement efforts and a baseline from which communities could measure improvement with periodic surveys. Structure measures in this zone can be particularly useful for crisis systems in early development–for example, whether mobile crisis teams are available 24/7, whether services are accessible in multiple languages, whether law enforcement receives Crisis Intervention Team training.

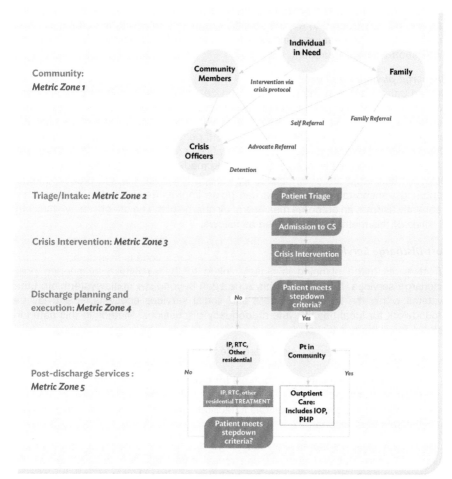

Fig. 3. Process-based metric framework. (*From* National Council for Mental Wellbeing. *Quality Measurement in Crisis Services*. Published online January 17, 2023. https://www.thenationalcouncil.org/resources/quality-measurement-in-crisis-services; with permission.)

Triage orintake

Does the triage function facilitate efficient entry into the appropriate intervention? Measures in this zone are the most well-developed in the crisis field and include many process measures of timeliness and efficiency such as the 988 Lifeline Performance Measures[13] (answer rate, abandonment rate, and average speed of answer), mobile crisis team measures (time from dispatch to arrival), and crisis stabilization facility measures based on established ED throughput measures (door to assessment time and left without being seen).[14] Metrics in this domain can also measure the effectiveness of triage processes. For example, when calls are diverted from 911 to 988, what percent are referred back to 911?

Crisis intervention

Is the intervention effective and expertly tailored to the patient's condition and circumstance? Effectiveness measures can include improvement in symptoms or function using standardized rating scales, measures on treatment outcome such as stabilization and reutilization rates, and patient reported outcomes such as satisfaction. Measures can also be constructed to ensure specific groups are receiving the care they need, for example, the percentage of individuals with an opiate use disorder who are offered medication-assisted treatment.

Discharge planning and execution

Did the patient arrive at the post-crisis service venue safe, without delay in service continuity, and able to participate in the services of the new venue? Process metrics can indicate whether key clinical steps occurred in preparing the patient for discharge (eg, percent with a completed safety plan, and percent with opiate use disorder discharged with naloxone), as well as administrative care coordination tasks (information transmitted to the next level care provider and medication reconciliation completion). Delays in discharge are often caused by transportation issues, and process metrics capturing transportation wait times can guide improvement efforts. Reutilization is frequently used as an outcome measure of discharge planning effectiveness; the complexities of this metric are discussed as follows.

Post-Discharge Services

Effective discharge planning is closely linked to the availability of needed post-discharge services. Measures in this zone span beyond the crisis system into other systems within the larger healthcare and social services ecosystems and lay the groundwork for local health system adequacy discussions. Metrics in this category ask the following questions.

- Are the available service slots adequate for the volume of crisis service discharge referrals?
- Is the service intensity array optimal for patient outcomes post-discharge from crisis services?
- Are specialized services available to facilitate optimal outcomes for crisis service patients post-discharge?

Commonly used measures like 7-day or 10-day follow-up begin to address these questions. More detailed analysis can reveal care gaps for specific groups; for example, tracking whether patients are admitted to higher levels of care because of a lack of lesser restrictive options or the percentage of patients in need of substance use disorder services who were successfully connected to the needed care. Such analyses often require retrospective chart review. Case Example 1 (**Box 1**) describes a process where this information could be captured in real-time.

A Person-Centered Framework for Crisis Metrics

In addition to monitoring how well a system is performing specific processes, metrics can also indicate whether a system is living up to its stated values. System values are defined with input from the customers and stakeholders discussed earlier including the people served, their families and loved ones, first responders, and other service providers with whom the crisis system collaborates. Then metrics are chosen to represent these values. One way to accomplish this is by using a quality improvement tool called a Critical-to-Quality tree,[15] which is designed to help an organization translate the "voice of the customer" into discrete measures. This approach has been used to create metrics specific to crisis facilities.[14] Here the authors apply this approach to the entire crisis system. This framework is outlined in **Fig. 4** and uses the mnemonic ACCESS TO HELP to describe a core set of values for crisis systems. Each value is defined in non-technical customer-focused language and mapped to example metrics.

Box 1
Case example 1: real-time measurement of the discharge planning process

Discharge, transfer, and post-discharge plans are critical in crisis services. Patients will need to leave crisis services at some point-even if not completely restored in functioning.

A process that is designed to review critical data in real-time around a potentially high-risk juncture can promote clarity in clinical reasoning. It can also draw attention to ecosystem gaps in a quantifiable way (because downstream resources are often the most critical factor in risk-acceptable discharge planning).

At the point of discharge, a critical milestone question might be: "Is the proposed aftercare plan adequate in light of the patient's symptoms, coping, risk of harm, and their access to community-based resources, such as living arrangements?

An engineering and process-design step in this context would be an automatic escalation process ("flag") that requires the team to pause, review or re-evaluate the situation and a "code" that requires the team to make alternative plans (including deploying additional resources) if significant discharge or transfer risk questions remain open. The Universal Protocol or "time out" performed in general medical settings to reduce medical errors is good example of an engineered protocol.

The automatic escalation is designed to assist ("flag") a situation "in the moment" for the treatment provider/team to assess the situation more closely, to determine whether the proposed disposition plan is optimal.

An example of a useful process metric would be to track the percentage of disposition plans that require a flag or a code for further review. This could assist the team in determining the effectiveness of the discharge planning process over time.

This approach complements the process-based approach, and the benefits of both approaches are fully realized when they are used together. Many of the metrics identified using the process-based approach are also included in the values-based approach. The values-based approach creates a framework to ensure that metrics related to each process zone are aligned to system values, creating a powerful tool to measure the performance of the system as a whole. Case Example 2 (**Box 2**) describes how Arizona has used this approach to develop comprehensive system measures aligned toward the system value of providing care in the least intrusive manner. Additionally, this approach identifies cross-cutting concepts such as equity and the need to stratify metrics by race and ethnicity across process zones and value domains in order to identify disparities.

Quality Measurement as a Catalyst for System Improvement and Transformation

It is hoped that outcome of a collective, multi-stakeholder, and person-centered approach to quality measurement is the adoption of transparent information-sharing and collaboration in service of iterative and continuous quality improvement (CQI) that moves the system closer to meeting its ideal values. Well-designed quality improvement programs focus on identifying opportunities for improvement (eg, flawed processes or workflows, and care gaps) rather than placing blame on individual performers within the systems. It is also important to set expectations: progress even in the best of circumstances will be incremental and at times tortuous because of the difficulties encountered by the populations experiencing significant crises.

First, Find the "Why"

While it can be tempting to jump straight to selecting or creating performance metrics for the healthcare ecosystem, it is important to begin by working collaboratively to

	Value	Meaning	Examples
A	**Accessible/ Affordable**	I am welcomed wherever I go. I am not turned away.	• Percentage of help-seekers who receive appropriate care vs. all who have sought care. • Percentage of persons seeking care who are turned away due to lack of coverage vs declined due to not being able to afford care.
C	**Collaborative**	Helpers work in partnership with me, my family, my caregivers, and other responders.	• The programs assess consumer/family satisfaction surveys and/or net promoter scores.
C	**Comprehensive**	I get help for all my issues that are part of the crisis.	• Access to medical screening. • Able to treat co-occurring substance use disorder (SUD), intellectual/developmental disorder (I/DD), etc.
E	**Equitable**	The quality of services I receive are not affected by my race, ethnicity, gender, sexual orientation, etc.	• Stratify outcome metrics (e.g., return to crisis centers, access to care) by race/ethnicity and other key demographics (e.g., ZIP code). What percentage of poor outcomes are disproportionately influenced by performance in underrepresented populations?
S	**Safe**	My experience of help is safe and not harmful. I am never traumatized by asking for help.	• What percentage of individuals presenting in crisis end up injured, hurt or killed while doing so?
S	**Successful**	The care I receive meets my needs.	• Readmission rates. • Symptom reduction.

	Value	Meaning	Examples
T	**Timely**	I get help quickly enough to meet my needs.	• Time to intervention (e.g., call answer times, mobile dispatch times, facility door-to-doctor times). • Abandonment rate (e.g., call abandonment, left without being seen, etc.). • Lag time between seeking care and receiving care.
O	**Ongoing**	I receive help to move from my crisis situation to ongoing support that wrap around me to help me thrive.	• Successful linkage to continuing care at adequate intensity: 3-, 7-, 30-, 60-, 90-day follow up.

	Value	Meaning	Examples
H	**Hopeful**	I am helped to feel more hopeful, and I make better decisions as a result.	• Decrease in suicide, violence, self-harm. • Personal Outcome Measures (POMS).
E	**Engaging**	I am treated as a valuable customer, with respect and dignity.	• Complaints, adverse incidents, escalation.
L	**Least Intrusive**	I receive help in a place that is designed to meet my needs.	• Avoidance of inappropriate emergency department use or arrest diversion, voluntary conversion.
P	**Publicized**	I know who to call and/or where to go.	• Information about call lines and walk in centers, increased use of 988 vs. 911.

Fig. 4. Person-centered metrics framework. (*From* National Council for Mental Wellbeing. *Quality Measurement in Crisis Services*. Published online January 17, 2023. https://www. thenationalcouncil.org/resources/quality-measurement-in-crisis-services; with permission.)

Box 2
Case example 2: Arizona's alignment of metrics toward common system values

Arizona has built a robust crisis system over the past several decades. The system is coordinated via the state Medicaid agency which braids funding from Medicaid, federal block grants, and other funds ensuring all individuals in need are served regardless of payer. The state contracts with a Regional Behavioral Health Authority (RBHA) in each geographic service area which in turn contract with individual service providers. The RBHA serves as the "accountable entity" and collects and integrates data from multiple sources, including the 988 crisis contact center, mobile crisis teams, and crisis stabilization facilities. This data is used for quality and operations management. A core value in the system is that individuals should have their crisis stabilized in the least-intrusive manner that is safely possible (the "L" in ACCESS TO HELP). To measure adherence to this value, all components of the crisis system (crisis line, mobile teams, facilities) report a variety of metrics that span all process zones to support their alignment toward this common goal.

- Community disposition: Each component has a metric that is defined as the percentage of encounters in which the person's crisis was resolved without having to escalate to a higher level of care (eg, crisis calls resolved without dispatching mobile crisis, mobile crisis encounters resolved without transport to an ED or crisis facility, crisis facility encounters resolved without admission to inpatient)
- Law enforcement involvement: crisis lines and mobile teams measure both the percentage of calls in which they request a law enforcement response (and work to reduce it), as well as how many calls they receive via processes designed to divert callers away from law enforcement responses (eg, 988/911 co-location)
- Involuntary commitment: Mobile crisis teams measure the percent of encounters resulting in an involuntary commitment, while crisis facilities measure the percent of involuntary individuals that were able to be engaged in their treatment and converted to voluntary status.

Crisis adjacent organizations track metrics supporting this value as well. For example, the Tucson Police Department measures the percentage of mental health transports, in which they were able to engage with the individual and transport them voluntarily without the use of involuntary commitment, and the City of Tucson measures the percentage of 911 calls diverted to the crisis line.

---

define system values. Values represent aspirations and desires (the "why") behind transformation efforts. While often unstated, values can be a powerful motivator for system change (or resistance to said change). Furthermore, having a clear set of values provides a framework for decision-making around selecting (or rejecting) specific metrics. Achieving alignment around a clear unified vision, codifying that vision through a carefully articulated value framework, and selecting metrics that track progress along achieving that vision can be extremely effective in sustaining buy-in through the inevitable setbacks that accompany any transformation effort. Investing time and effort up front to define values and to bring all stakeholders into alignment can be a critical first step toward sustained system change.

The first step is to convene a stakeholder group with representation of all users and stakeholders. The convening body could be a government agency (eg, state, county, or local behavioral health authority), payer (eg, managed Medicaid), or community collaborative such as newly developing 988 advisory or crisis coordinating committees. The *Roadmap to the Ideal Crisis System* report[16] includes more details on the importance of accountable entities and community collaboratives with strategies for creating them.

Once the right stakeholders are at the table, the next step is to define and memorialize the system's values, goals, and intended results. These will serve as a foundation and framework for the system's definition of quality benchmarks. All of the process zones and value domains discussed in this article are parts of a comprehensive crisis system, but different communities will prioritize them differently based on their history, culture, strengths, and gaps. For example, a community that has been plagued with long waiting lists might prioritize values and processes related to rapid access to care, while a community that recently suffered a traumatic event such as a police-involved death might prioritize processes and values related to least intrusive care that minimizes law enforcement involvement.

The next steps involve mapping the current and ideal states so that gaps can be identified. This includes an inventory of existing crisis services and supports within the ecosystem and mapping how individuals flow through the system. Once there is consensus an understanding of how the current system works, the next step is to map the ideal operational flow and patient treatment pathways through both the Crisis System and the Healthcare Ecosystem (logic models can be very effective in this strategic stage.). This exercise will help the group assess current gaps, both in terms of how people flow through the system and whether the processes are meeting system values.

The learnings from this work can then be used to develop metrics using the process-based and values-based frameworks described earlier. These metrics provide the foundation for establishing achievable improvement goals that are specific, measurable, actionable, realistic, and time-bound as in Case Example 3 (**Box 3**).

Systemwide Approaches to Performance Improvement

The authors have described frameworks for defining crisis system metrics and how this approach helps align the multiple processes and components of the system toward common goals. This provides a foundation for systems to identify areas needing improvement and work together to improve performance.

Box 3
Case example 3: Philadelphia's crisis transformation

Philadelphia's Crisis System Transformation has garnered national attention. In July 2022, Philadelphia was selected to host the federal launch of 988, in recognition of its efforts. While the adult crisis system transformation was catalyzed by the shooting death of Walter Wallace in October 2020, the groundwork began in the summer of 2019. It began with the convening of internal and external stakeholder groups. As the project team studied advanced Crisis systems across the country, a series of conversations elucidated the concerns of various stakeholders, including service-recipients, families, crisis-system service providers, law enforcement and other allied city services and agencies.

One key finding from these discussions was that Philadelphia's crisis system relied heavily on coercive measures such as Emergency Involuntary Treatment orders (colloquially referred to as "302s" in Philadelphia). A review of 302 data showed that this tactic was disproportionately applied to communities and individuals of color. Additionally, stakeholders described the 302 experiences as often being traumatizing to the service recipient.

As a result of these discussions, Philadelphia's stakeholders elucidated well-defined, and specific values and clear goals that have guided transformation efforts. They are.
1. Reduced law enforcement involvement in behavioral health crisis.
2. Reduced involuntary commitments (302).
3. Reduction in acute care service utilization and length of stay in acute care settings.
4. Increased crisis resolution in the community with family and social supports.
5. Increased warm handoff to community-based programs and services that address social determinants of health.
6. Increased individual, family, and community satisfaction with the crisis response.

All stakeholders should participate in quality improvement initiatives but they may focus on different metrics depending on their role in the ecosystem. Metrics for payers, counties, or other high level "accountable entities" are more systemic while metrics for individual service providers have a narrower scope. This is because to be actionable, metrics must measure a process that is within the sphere of influence of the organization to improve.

For example, a system may decide to focus on the value "Ongoing" which is defined from the person-centered perspective as: "I receive help to move from my crisis situation to ongoing support that wraps around me to help me thrive." The suggested system metric (percentage of patients who received outpatient follow-up within 7 days of their crisis encounter) is a commonly used HEDIS measure and appropriate for an accountable entity such as managed care organization that is in a position to influence the behavior of its contracted service providers. The providers, however, should choose metrics more narrowly focused on parts of the processes performed by their staff in zone 4 (discharge planning) and zone 5 (post-discharge services). For example, the referring crisis provider might measure percent of discharges with a documented follow-up appointment and other measures of care coordination such as whether information was sent to the receiving clinic. Additionally, as in Case Example 1 (see **Box 1**), real-time measurement and automated flags can built into the EHR to identify when these processes are not being performed so they can be addressed in real-time. Conversely, the receiving clinic might implement measures showing the availability of appointments within the 7-day timeframe, whether they called the patient before the appointment for a reminder or outreach, how long individuals wait in the waiting room,and so forth.

Accountable entities responsible for oversight and payment have an important role to play in collectively improving performance. By linking incentive payments to these measures, payers can influence crisis providers and clinics to focus on processes that lead to a better 7-day follow-up. By convening multistakeholder collaboratives, they can bring the components of the system together to share and discuss performance data and collaboratively work on solutions using quality improvement (QI) methods such as Plan-Do-Study-Act cycles. Solutions may involve both involve internal QI work at the provider level and also action by the accountable entity itself, such as funding new services to fill identified gaps in care like post-discharge peer navigation or developing software to improve the appointment-making process.

The Complexity of Ecosystem-Wide Measurement

Crisis services are among the most intersectional areas of health care, with interfaces between emergency and mental health specialty call centers, emergency medical services, mobile crisis teams, police and jails, clinics, schools, health systems, and many other agencies.

Determining how well the authors are serving their clients goes beyond defining metrics using existing data—the authors must consider novel approaches to linking data systems to strengthen informatics opportunities. Measuring the performance of a crisis system requires a robust ability to share, aggregate, and manage information across multiple types of providers. Best practices for linkages include matching along key identifiers (name, date of birth, and social security number), though these data are rarely collected in full by call centers. Therefore, systems need to implement call-specific IDs that bridge data systems to facilitate retrospective linkages that can traverse call center, mobile unit, health system, and criminal justice data systems. Fortunately, recent and pending changes to Health Insurance Portability and Accountability Act (1996), 42 Code of Federal Regulations Part 2, and Office of the National

Coordinator for Health Information Technology or CMS interoperability will make sharing information more feasible and efficient.

Such approaches allow for going beyond performance measures like response times and get into more meaningful process measures (eg, post-crisis routine care utilization, post-crisis acute or crisis care reutilization, post-crisis arrest or jail entry, and so forth.), as well as actual outcomes (all-cause morbidity or mortality, housing status, patient-reported outcomes).

Interpreting such measures can be a complex task. Reutilization, for example, may be interpreted as a negative outcome because the crisis service was unable to divert from higher intensity care settings, but at the same time, people in crisis should be encouraged to seek help for appropriate reasons (eg, worsening symptoms or risky behaviors). Similarly, consider the increasingly common metric Hospital Diversion Rate, which measures the percentage visits that result in a disposition other than inpatient admission. An optimal rate of inpatient hospital diversion is unknown and depends on many factors, including the ability of the healthcare ecosystem to wrap around and engage with the patient after a crisis encounter. Another important consideration is the impact of the length of time to bring symptoms under control. A crisis system that considers diversion from inpatient hospitalization in the absence of longitudinal data on the functional outcomes of patients diverted may result in a false sense of success. There is a need to understand at a population level what a "reasonable" benchmark rate is for these key outcomes. Furthermore, service providers may adopt practices akin to cherry-picking, in which certain groups are excluded from engaging with services, and thus, result in inflated performance on certain metrics. Risk-adjustment funding and models of care demonstrating effectiveness in these more complex populations should reduce exclusionary practices across the ecosystem.

Finally, equity must be an essential aim for crisis services measurement. To understand potential disparities in delivery of crisis care, it is necessary to routinely collect relevant demographic data such as gender identity, sexual orientation, race, ethnicity, and language preferences. Reporting of metrics outcomes should be stratified by subgroups to allow for identification of disparities and when found, monitoring should ensure that remedies are effective at advancing equity in service delivery—both internal to the crisis service delivery and in the customization of broad ecosystem resources and solutions.

SUMMARY

Measuring the quality of care in crisis systems is no easy task. Fortunately, multiple approaches are available to systems that seek to ensure high-quality and person-centered, equitable delivery of crisis care. Whether using conventional or more person-centered approaches, systems can benefit from overcoming barriers to measurement and ensuring that they are employing continuous quality improvement practices to improve crisis care for all.

CLINICS CARE POINTS

- Quality measures can be a powerful tool to align the parts of a crisis system toward common goals based on a shared set of values.
- System engineering methods provide a framework to both define measures and also build safety checkpoints to ensure key processes are performed correctly and consistently.
- Metrics should be meaningful, feasible, and actionable with well-defined measure specifications.

- All stakeholders should participate in quality improvement initiatives but they may focus on different metrics depending on their role in the ecosystem.
- To improve health equity, it is necessary to routinely collect relevant demographic data such as gender identity, sexual orientation, race, ethnicity, and language preferences. Measures should be stratified by sub-groups to identify disparities.

DISCLOSURE

J. Parks is consultant to Boehringer-Ingelheim. B. Shaw is an employee of the United States Department of Health and Human Services Substance Abuse and Mental Health Services Administration. This article does not represent an official position or opinion of the United States Department of Health and Human Services. Other authors have nothing to disclose.

REFERENCES

1. National Council for Mental Wellbeing, Quality measurement in crisis services, Available at: https://www.thenationalcouncil.org/resources/quality-measurement-in-crisis-services/, 2023, Accessed January 22, 2024.
2. Nundy S, Cooper LA, Mate KS. The quintuple aim for health care improvement: a new imperative to advance health equity. JAMA 2022;327(6):521.
3. Wu J, Wang Y, Tao L, et al. Stakeholders in the healthcare service ecosystem. Procedia CIRP 2019;83:375–9.
4. Donabedian A. An introduction to quality Assurance in health care. New York: Oxford University Press; 2003.
5. Cella D, Hahn EA, Jensen SE, et al. Patient-reported outcomes in performance measurement, Available at: https://www.ncbi.nlm.nih.gov/books/NBK424378/, 2015, Accessed January 22, 2024.
6. Hermann RC, Palmer RH. Common ground: a framework for selecting core quality measures for mental health and substance abuse care. PS 2002;53(3):281–7.
7. Hettinger AZ, Roth EM, Bisantz AM. Cognitive engineering and health informatics: Applications and intersections. J Biomed Inf 2017;67:21–33.
8. O'Neill SM, Clyne B, Bell M, et al. Why do healthcare professionals fail to escalate as per the early warning system (EWS) protocol? A qualitative evidence synthesis of the barriers and facilitators of escalation. BMC Emerg Med 2021; 21(1):15.
9. Centers for Medicare & Medicaid Services, Measure specification, Available at: https://mmshub.cms.gov/measure-lifecycle/measure-specification/overview, 2023, Accessed January 22, 2024.
10. Partnership for Quality Measurement, Repository measure database, Available at: https://p4qm.org/measures, Accessed January 22, 2024.
11. National Center for Quality Assurance, HEDIS and performance measurement, Available at: https://www.ncqa.org/hedis/, Accessed January 22, 2024.
12. Velázquez T., Most U.S. adults remain unaware of 988 suicide and crisis lifeline, Available at: https://www.pewtrusts.org/en/research-and-analysis/articles/2023/05/23/most-us-adults-remain-unaware-of-988-suicide-and-crisis-lifeline, 2023, Accessed January 22, 2024.
13. Substance Abuse and Mental Health Services Administration, 988 lifeline performance metrics, Available at: https://www.samhsa.gov/find-help/988/performance-metrics, Accessed January 22, 2024.

14. Balfour ME, Tanner K, Jurica PJ, et al. Crisis reliability indicators supporting emergency services (CRISES): a framework for developing performance measures for behavioral health crisis and psychiatric emergency programs. Community Ment Health J 2016;52(1):1–9.
15. Hessing T., Critical to quality tree (CTQ). Six Sigma Study Guide, Available at: https://sixsigmastudyguide.com/critical-to-quality-tree/, 2018. Accessed January 22, 2024.
16. National Council for Mental Wellbeing. Roadmap to the Ideal Crisis System: Essential Elements, Measurable Standards and Best Practices for Behavioral Health Crisis Response, 2021, Available at: http://www.thenationalcouncil.org/resources/roadmap-to-the-ideal-crisis-system/. Accessed January 22, 2024.

The Crisis Continuum

The Journey Toward 988
A Historical Perspective on Crisis Hotlines in the United States

John Draper, PhD[a],*, Richard T. McKeon, PhD, MPH[b]

KEYWORDS

- Suicide prevention • Crisis • Hotline • Lifeline • 988 • Crisis chat • Crisis text

KEY POINTS

- In the twentieth century, community crisis and suicide prevention efforts were not integrated into community mental health care systems. Rather, behavioral health crises were primarily managed either through public safety response systems or anonymous crisis hotlines.
- At the beginning of the twenty-first century, the Substance Abuse and Mental Health Services Administration (SAMHSA) grant-funded the networking, certification, and evaluation of crisis hotlines. This effort led to the establishment of the National Suicide Prevention Lifeline and the first definitive evidence of the efficacy of crisis hotlines in reducing emotional distress and suicidality in service users. The evaluations also showed the need for more uniform, evidence-based standards, trainings, and practices across the network of centers throughout the 50 states.
- Increasing public awareness and the use of the toll-free Lifeline service—as well as evidence of the service's effectiveness—led to the overall growth and expansion of Lifeline-related services nationwide. The Department of Veterans Affairs (VA) established and integrated the Veterans Crisis Line into the Lifeline network number, and national helpline services were extended via the Lifeline Crisis Chat and Text services, as well as the SAMHSA-funded Disaster Distress Helpline.
- The continuing increase in suicide rates inspired Congress to propose in 2018 the consideration of a national 3-digit number to enable greater access to the Lifeline's 10-digit-dial service. After careful study of reports from SAMHSA and the VA, as well as inputs from a wide variety of stakeholders nationally, the US Federal Communications Commission assigned a new 3-digit number to the Lifeline in 2020, "988.".
- The establishment of 988 holds the promise of transforming behavioral health and crisis care in America's twenty-first century, by providing a complete public health response (instead of solely a public safety response) to behavioral health crises, as well as integrating the primary value of access to care "anywhere, for anyone at any time" into traditional behavioral health care systems.

[a] Behavioral Health Link, Inc, 7423 Narrows Avenue, Brooklyn, NY 11209, USA; [b] Center for Mental Health Services, SAMHSA, 988 and Behavioral Health Crisis Coordinating Office, 5600 Fishers Ln, Rockville, MD 20852, USA
* Corresponding author. 1201 Peachtree Street, NE Building, 400 Suite 1215, Atlanta, GA 30361.
E-mail address: jdraper@ihrcorp.com

Psychiatr Clin N Am 47 (2024) 473–490
https://doi.org/10.1016/j.psc.2024.04.003
0193-953X/24/© 2024 Elsevier Inc. All rights are reserved, including those for text and data mining, AI training, and similar technologies.

When the US Federal Communications Commission (FCC) recommended the designation of 988 as the national 3-digit dialing code for suicide and behavioral health crisis in 2019, they cited an expectation that it would "help increase the effectiveness of suicide prevention efforts, ease access to crisis services, reduce the stigma surrounding suicide and mental health conditions, and ultimately save lives."[1] In a report to Congress prior to 988's national launch on July 16, 2022, the US Substance Abuse and Mental Health Services Administration (SAMHSA) noted that 988 would spur behavioral health systems transformation like 911 has catalyzed change in US emergency medical services.[2] That report described how 988 was also intended to reduce unnecessary encounters of persons in behavioral health crisis with both the police and hospital emergency departments.

The 988 number has become the more public face of the National Suicide Prevention Lifeline (Lifeline), a network of locally and independently operated crisis hotline centers (eg, "crisis centers"), a project that has been funded by the SAMHSA since 2001. This network's role as the nation's front door and safety net for suicide prevention, crisis, and mental health services is the result of a historical trajectory for crisis hotlines in the United States. In the 60 years of their existence, crisis hotlines frequently emerged as a "grassroots" community resource designed to be *an alternative* to accessing traditional mental health services. For us to understand how 988 may transform behavioral health systems in America, it is important to understand how crisis hotlines have also evolved over these many decades, and how they may ultimately affect how people seek and receive effective behavioral health care in the United States.

BRIEF HISTORY OF CRISIS AND SUICIDE PREVENTION HOTLINES IN THE UNITED STATES

Throughout the twentieth century, in the United States, custodial approaches—law enforcement and institutionalization—were the primary means for communities responding to individuals experiencing mental health and suicidal crises.[3,4] As public safety responses reinforced the long-standing stigma and discrimination associated with mental health crises, crisis hotlines began to spring up in the mid-twentieth century as an alternative means for people in crisis to seek help. A crisis service that was free, anonymous, and 24/7/365—and accessible in the privacy of one's home—ran counter to the hours-limited, inconvenient, expensive, and nonanonymous offerings available (or not) in community mental health clinics. Importantly, the anonymity of early hotlines allowed people in crisis to access help with less fear of police intervention.

The Los Angeles Suicide Prevention Center

In 1958, a National Institute of Mental Health grant allowed psychologists Ed Shneidman and Norman Farberow along with psychiatrist Robert Litman to establish the Los Angeles Suicide Prevention Center (LASPC), the first of its kind in the United States. The LASPC was originally focused on the evaluation and treatment of survivors of suicide attempts in hospitals when word-of-mouth about the center prompted persons in suicidal crisis to call the service at all hours.[5] In 1962, the LASPC piloted a 24/7/365 hotline service with clinicians responding, soon staffing the 24/7 line with volunteers as a more practical alternative. LASPC volunteers established rapport, assessed for safety, and collaborated with callers on a "treatment plan." LASPC was the first crisis center to collect data about anonymous callers' problems, demographics, and history of past suicidality and treatment.[5] Through the LASPC, research and clinical practices related to suicidality became integrated with hotline services.

By 1971, over 200 crisis centers were operating, with 1 expert proclaiming that each of the centers owed a debt to LASPC for developing their "basic concepts of suicide prevention."[6] LASPC's co-director, Ed Shneidman, founded the American Association of Suicidology (AAS) in 1968, which became a global hub for suicide prevention research and began accrediting crisis centers in best practices in 1976.[7] In addition, the use of nonprofessionals and volunteers at the LASPC and many other crisis centers gained considerable notice. Suicide prevention expert Louis Dublin described the use of nonprofessionals as "the single most important discovery in the 50-year history of the suicide prevention movement."[8]

Crisis Hotlines and Behavioral Health Systems in the Late Twentieth Century

While the use of volunteers on hotlines was good news for 24/7 clinical workforce challenges, it created a persistent perception that suicide prevention was the province of paraprofessionally staffed hotlines, while community clinical services were designed for ongoing "non-crisis" treatment. Consequently, when hotlines could not de-escalate suicidal crises over the phone, the default venue for clinically managing psychiatric crises became hospital emergency departments into the 1990s.[9] To this extent, calls to 911 for psychiatric emergency transport to hospitals typically prompted a police response, further reinforcing the public safety approaches long familiar to persons in behavioral health crisis in America.

By 1990s, several metropolitan areas around the country were beginning to utilize crisis services as a primary means for connecting people to care in their behavioral health system. SAMHSA's new Center for Mental Health Services conducted a survey of 69 well-developed crisis care systems, with crisis hotlines delineated as an essential element of more advanced crisis systems, along with mobile crisis outreach teams and community crisis receiving facilities.[10] While most crisis centers surveyed indicated telephone counseling and information and referral as a function, nearly all underscored their primary concern was to screen and assess callers for face-to-face services. At this time, there was no clear evidence that crisis hotlines themselves were effective in reducing suicidality or emotional distress with the people they served.[11]

SUBSTANCE ABUSE AND MENTAL HEALTH SERVICES ADMINISTRATION GRANT TO NETWORK AND CERTIFY CRISIS HOTLINES

In 2001, congressional funding was provided to SAMHSA to establish a national network of crisis hotlines, linked to a single toll-free number, to effectively reach and serve all persons at risk of suicide across the United States.[12] The grant administrator's "networking and certifying" objectives included

- Building a network infrastructure of independently operated and funded local crisis call centers in every state. Calls to a national toll-free line would be connected to providers nearest to the caller, based on the area code they were calling from.
- A national accrediting body such as AAS would certify this coast-to-coast network of local crisis hotlines, to further establish base line expectations of member center services.
- National best practices for crisis centers would be identified through ongoing evaluations conducted by an independent team of researchers funded through the grant.

In 2004, SAMHSA awarded the hotline grant to the New York City (NYC)–based organization Vibrant Emotional Health (or Vibrant, formerly known as the Mental Health

Association of NYC). Vibrant and its long-time partners, the National Association of State Mental Health Program Directors (NASMHPD), successfully launched the new 1-800-273-TALK (8255) service with 109 network members in January 2005. That same year, Vibrant established 3 national advisory committees that would build field consensus on best approaches for reaching and serving people in suicidal crisis: the Steering Committee; the Consumer-Survivor (persons with lived experience of suicide loss and suicide attempts) Committee; and the Standards, Trainings and Practices Committee (STPC) (researchers, program evaluators, crisis center directors, and so forth).

LIFELINE EVALUATION FINDINGS

Perhaps the most influential requirement at the conception of the SAMHSA hotline grant was dedicating network center participation to ongoing evaluation efforts to continuously improve crisis services. In the first 20 years of the grant, 68 network centers participated in 15 studies published in peer-reviewed journals. The published works and **Fig. 1** illustrate the iterative process through which Lifeline center practices are implemented, evaluated, and refined to continuously improve service quality. The findings from these evaluations of crisis hotlines have proven to be groundbreaking for the field of suicide prevention and crisis hotlines, both nationally and internationally.[13]

SAMHSA-funded investigations of network member hotlines consisted of mostly discerning caller outcomes associated with counselor behaviors. **Table 1** comprises a sample of early Lifeline evaluations where inbound caller outcomes were reported by the users themselves. Most evaluations were overseen by Dr Madelyn Gould and her team from the Research Foundation for Mental Health at Columbia's Psychiatric Institute.

As noted in **Table 1**, all evaluations observed positive outcomes for callers, with most demonstrating significant reductions in both suicidal and crisis states for service users.[14–17] Brian Mishara and his evaluation team from Quebec[16] underscored 2 areas of counselor practices that were associated with these positive outcomes. First, counselors need to establish good contact/rapport with callers. Second, they found that "active listening" alone was insufficient for effectively reducing suicidal distress; some degree of guiding the conversation and collaborating with the caller to address his/her concerns was essential ("collaborative problem solving").

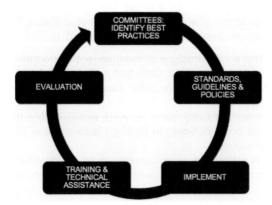

Fig. 1. Lifeline iterative process for developing evidence-based national network standards, practices, and policies.

Table 1
Substance Abuse and Mental Health Services Administration–funded evaluations of networked crisis centers, outcomes, and impact

PI & Date of Evaluation Publication	Purpose of Evaluation	Key Outcomes & Recommendations	Program Impact
Gould & Kalafat, 2007 Kalafat & Gould, 2007	Post-call crisis and suicidal outcomes (end of call and follow-up, at approx. 3 wk), 1085 suicidal callers. Post-call crisis outcomes (end of call and follow-up), 1617 crisis callers.	• Is reaching seriously suicidal people (callers with suicide plans, attempts, and so forth). • Reductions in crisis and suicidal states by end of call and at follow-up. • 11.7% of callers not assessed for suicide • Need to follow-up with callers still at risk (43% post-call).	• Justified continued increases in federal funding of Lifeline services. • Led to SAMHSA-funded follow-up grants to Lifeline centers. • Influenced need for developing national suicide risk assessment standards.
Mishara et al, 2007	Silent monitoring of 2611 callers to 14 network crisis centers to determine what counselor processes affect caller outcomes.	• Centers vary greatly in helper behaviors. • Some lives may have been saved. • Need to train and reinforce empathy, respect, and collaborative problem-solving for good outcomes. • Many counselors did not assess risk and/ or did not fully assess risk.	• Influenced need to standardize risk assessment framework for all centers in network. • Led to Lifeline sponsoring ASIST trainings for network and later developing a uniform training for all network counselors in 2022.
Gould et al, 2013	To assess impact of Lifeline-sponsored ASIST on counselor behaviors at 17 centers. Silently monitored 1507 exchanges between suicidal callers and ASIST-trained counselors.	• Callers working with ASIST-trained counselors felt less depressed and suicidal and more hopeful by the end of the call • Distinct behaviors from ASIST having an impact: exploring caller reasons for living and their informal supports.	• Led to continued Lifeline support of ASIST trainings at network centers. • Later incorporated effective counselor behaviors into Lifeline online best practice trainings for all network counselors in 2022.

Partial summary of key evaluation findings published 2007 to 2021.
Abbreviation: ASIST, applied suicide intervention skills training.

These findings were unprecedented in clearly demonstrating the impact that crisis lines had on reducing caller distress and suicidality. Since 1990s, crisis lines had been trending toward focusing more on their screening, assessment, and referral function, with the belief that care and treatment for people in crisis was best performed in face-to-face clinical settings. In contrast, the findings of the Gould, Kalafat, and Mishara teams indicated that the assessment and referral functions of these hotlines needed considerable attention, while the potential for crisis lines as a "mental health service" was much greater than had been previously known.

Although these initial evaluation findings answered many long-standing questions about hotline efficacy and related practices, each discerned several marked short-comings in counselor practices that required systematic attention. In all, findings from these studies identified 3 major areas as targets for practice improvement: the need for uniform standards and practices for *suicide risk assessment* among callers; a clear policy for necessary actions to take to maintain the safety of callers assessed to be at *imminent risk (IR)* of suicide; and a need for *follow-up* with callers at risk, to both de-escalate risk and promote linkages to community care.[13]

NATIONAL STANDARDS AND PRACTICES

Toward developing consensus approaches to actualize the 3 main recommendations emerging from the initial SAMHSA-funded hotline evaluations, the Lifeline formed in 2005 a national advisory group now referred to as the STPC. The STPC included project evaluators and other leading suicide prevention researchers, practitioners, and crisis center directors from around the country. Following are among the most prominent standards, guidelines, and practices that ultimately emerged from the ongoing evaluation findings and committee recommendations.

National Suicide Risk Assessment Standards for Crisis Hotlines

To better assure that all callers to the National Suicide Prevention Lifeline would be appropriately assessed for suicidality, Vibrant required all network member centers to adopt their STPC-approved standards for assessing risk beginning in 2007, with a recently updated edition in 2022. Rather than venturing to develop or identify a specific risk assessment instrument where reliability and validity would be questionable, the Lifeline's STPC instead chose to create a standard framework for suicide risk assessment.[18]

This framework was shaped around 4 core principles of risk assessment, distinguished by the committee's factor analysis from various crisis center risk assessment scales and decades of research in suicide assessment. Three of Lifeline's 4 principles are consistent with STPC Chair Thomas Joiner's Interpersonal Theory of Suicide[19] which proposes that the combination of suicidal desire with intent and acquired capability is associated with the risk of suicide. Buffers–the fourth core principle– relate to established protective factors that can moderate or mitigate against suicidal desire or intent. What factors indicate each of these principal areas of suicide assessment and how they interact to affect potential safety concerns are described in **Table 2**.

The Lifeline's STPC underscored in 2007 that suicide risk assessment was not intended to predict suicidal behavior. Rather, it is intended to help counselors collaborate with callers in care planning, to explore "the most effective way to reduce callers' isolation, anxiety, and despair, and to begin the exploration of alternative ways of addressing their problems."[18] This intention was further emphasized by Vibrant in their updated "Safety Assessment" standards in 2019.[20]

Table 2
988 suicide and crisis lifeline suicide risk assessment framework

Risk Principle	Indicators of Risk Principle[a]	Risk Principle Interactions Affecting Risk Ranges

Desire for suicide	Suicidal thoughts, often driven by feelings of hopelessness; feeling trapped and a burden to others, feeling intolerably alone, self-hatred, and intense psychological pain.	Low to moderate risk range
		• Suicidal desire or capability alone are present
		• Buffers against suicide are:
		  ○ Present to potentially reduce risk
		  ○ Absent to potentially enhance risk

Intent to die by suicide	Suicide attempt in progress, or suicide plan, including preparatory behaviors with an expressed intent to die.	Moderate to high risk range
		• Suicidal desire and intent are present
		• Suicidal desire and capability are present
		• Buffers against suicide are
		  ○ Present to potentially reduce risk
		  ○ Absent to potentially enhance risk

Capability for suicide	One's degree of fearlessness in taking suicidal actions, such as past suicide attempts and/or self-harming behaviors (eg, "practicing" to overcome fears of dying). Also includes available means and one's inability to control suicidal impulses (eg, emotional dysregulation, current intoxication, substance use, acute mental illness symptoms, and so forth). May also include history of violence and/or exposure to another's suicide.	High-risk range • Suicidal desire, intent, and capability are all present. • Buffers are not likely to mitigate risk
Buffers preventing suicide	Risk mitigating factors, such as having reasons for living, expressed ambivalence about dying, access to immediate social supports, future plans, engagement with the counselor, and personally held values against suicide.	

[a] Bolded indicators represent items with highest weight of research regarding contribution to risk, see *Vibrant Suicide Safety Policy 2022* and *Joiner et al, SLTB, 2007.*

Lifeline's efforts to improve risk assessment and collaboration with callers were encouraged by subsequent evaluations, including research reported by Rand on California-based crisis centers. The Rand findings demonstrated that callers to Lifeline member centers were much more likely to be assessed for suicide risk and feel less distressed by the end of the call than callers contacting non–Lifeline crisis centers.[21]

National Policy for Helping Callers at Imminent Risk of Suicide

Following the identification of a suicide assessment framework, the Lifeline STPC set out to identify best practices for counselors working with callers to be assessed at imminent risk of suicide (eg, "IR").[13]

Lifeline's policy noted that counselor actions to help callers at IR of suicide must consider least invasive approaches to preserve a caller's safety.[22] Less invasive approaches essentially ordain the need for committed *collaboration*, beginning with the counselor's collaboration with the caller to take actions to reduce their own risk ("active engagement"). These active collaborations extend to (a) supervisory consultation as needed and (b) center relationships with community crisis and emergency services that could respond to their callers to keep them safe. As a last resort, if the individual was *in the act of killing themselves* and/or is *unwilling or unable* to take actions to prevent their imminent suicide, the counselor would be compelled to activate emergency services ("active rescue," a 911 contact) on behalf of the caller's safety.

Table 3 provides examples of behaviors outlined by Lifeline's Policy to Help Callers at Imminent Risk of Suicide, which was recently updated by Vibrant in 2022 to underscore needs for active engagement and least invasive interventions.[23] It is important to note in the new policy edition that Vibrant has replaced the term "active rescue" to its more accurate label, "involuntary emergency service" activation, to distinguish it from consensual emergency services and all other collaborative means used by counselors to keep callers safe.

An evaluation of the policy's impact on Lifeline counselor behavior with callers at IR was undertaken.[24] Evaluators had previously estimated from samples that around 1 in 4 Lifeline callers presented suicide-related issues, with persons at highest (or "imminent") risk being a smaller subset of callers.[2] In reviewing 491 imminent risk calls, crisis counselors actively engaged the callers in collaborating to keep themselves safe on 76.4% of calls, providing an array of successful interventions ranging from safety planning, offering follow-up, engaging third-party support, or making mobile crisis referrals. Emergency rescue services, without the callers' collaboration, were needed on 24.6% of calls. These "active rescues" were largely limited to calls where callers expressed many or strong reasons for dying and had little sense of purpose in their lives. Having an attempt in progress, being intoxicated at the time of the call, and a low level of engagement with the crisis counselor also increased the odds of active rescue. Overall, findings indicated that the IR policy had a marked impact on improving counselor active engagement interventions with IR callers. For all calls to the Lifeline (including non-suicidal crises and information and referral needs), Vibrant reported that approximately 2% required a need for emergency services.[2]

Promotion of Follow-Up Contacts to Further Reduce Suicide Risk

As evaluators showed that some number of suicidal callers remained at risk after the initial call, Lifeline provided resources and guidelines to promote crisis center follow-up for callers at risk. Follow-up approaches ranging from hospitals sending post-discharge caring letters and postcards to persons who had been admitted for suicidality,[25,26] as well as follow-up calls and visits post-discharge[27,28] consistently demonstrated reductions in suicide attempts and deaths.

In 2008, SAMHSA began to provide Lifeline centers with funding specifically aimed at establishing follow-up services for high-risk Lifeline callers (later to include

Table 3
988 Lifeline policy for helping callers at imminent risk of suicide

Policy Intervention Area	Counselor or Center Behaviors	Related Interventions and Protocols
Active engagement	Intensive collaboration with caller to explore least invasive interventions to maintain safety and reduce risk. Empower caller choices that prevent their suicide, leveraging their resources and strengths.	Listening to caller's reasons for dying and engage reasons for living; safety planning, including removing access to lethal means, engaging immediate supports, coping strategies, attain agreement to receive urgent assistance (mobile crisis, voluntary transport to emergency room, and so forth)
Involuntary emergency intervention (*prev. "active rescue"*)	If active engagement efforts fail and person is unwilling and/or unable to choose actions that could reduce their imminent risk (including attempts in progress), counselor must initiate contact with emergency services to prevent the caller's suicide.	Utilize caller's available identifying information (caller ID, url address if chat, and so forth), share essential info with emergency officials to locate them and assure their safety. Track emergency service disposition and transport of individual, sharing information to authorities in support of individual's care and safety, where needed.
Community engagement and collaboration with crisis & emergency services	Network centers must investigate and promote alternatives to 911 interventions in their community. Develop relationships, cross-trainings, policies, and communications protocols with community first responder entities toward assuring optimal chain of care.	Center develops formal agreements, protocols, and trainings with first responder entities. Includes memorandums of understanding (MOUs)/protocols designed with mobile crisis teams, 911 public-safety answering points (PSAPs), local law enforcement, emergency medical service (EMS), emergency departments (EDs) and other receiving facilities, and so forth.

Extracted from 988 Suicide and Crisis Lifeline Safety Policy, Vibrant, 12/27/2022

local emergency department discharges).[13] To date, 44 follow-up grants to 41 crisis centers have been issued. For crisis centers, follow-up is usually by telephone and typically occurs between 24 and 48 hours after the initial contact. Phone calls are brief, and while they can be tailored to the individual's need, they are structured and focus on continued assessment of risk and safety, review and revision of the established safety plan, status of any upcoming appointments, and problem-solving obstacles to linkage. Follow-up typically continues until a caller is connected to care, is determined to be stable, and no longer in need of support or refuses services.

As with other Lifeline initiatives, follow-up practice within the network has been thoroughly evaluated by researchers. Initial findings indicate significant benefits, with 79.6% of callers indicating that the crisis center follow-up intervention stopped them from killing themselves, whereas 91% reported that it kept them safe.[29] Individuals who presented with higher levels of risk at the time of their initial call to the Lifeline perceived the follow-up intervention to be more valuable than those at lower suicide risk. Counselor activities, such as discussing distractors identified in the caller's safety plan, social contacts to call for help, and continued exploration of a caller's reasons for dying, were also found to be particularly helpful.

Lifeline follow-up evaluations established another major milestone for crisis hotlines. While AAS accreditation standards had long underscored the important function of following up with suicidal callers, most hotlines have been funded to focus on managing inbound calls. Gould's 2007 findings demonstrated the need for post-call follow-up to reduce suicidality and promote care linkages, and her subsequent evaluations of SAMHSA-follow-up- grant funded centers showed that such dedicated practices are essential to potentially saving lives.[13]

LIFELINE NETWORK EXPANSION BEFORE 988

Spurred by evaluations showing the Lifeline's effectiveness, federal and national stakeholders continued to build on the service. In 2006, Lifeline launched a specialized service option for Spanish language callers to the service in 2006, followed by the Veteran Administration's Veterans Crisis Line (VCL) in 2007 for current and past members of military service ("press 1"). Approximately 1 of every 4 callers to the Lifeline pressed 1 for assistance in the VCL's first decade.[13] Similar to the evaluation findings for the Lifeline, analyses of VCL's efficacy in serving callers found significant reductions in caller distress and suicidality during the call.[30]

Crisis Chat and Text Services

As online help-seeking became ubiquitous in the twenty-first century, some crisis centers began to venture into providing digital assistance to supplement their telephonic offerings. The VCL established the first federally funded crisis chat service in 2009, and the Lifeline followed suit in 2013. Individuals seeking crisis chat assistance could access help through the respective Web sites for each service. While the VCL added a text service in 2012, the Crisis Text Line (CTL) launched their broadly promoted national service in 2013 independent of the Lifeline. The CTL eventually joined the Lifeline when 988 integrated broad-scale text capabilities in 2022.

As with hotlines, evaluations of digital helplines showed considerable promise. Dr Gould's team evaluated both the Lifeline chat and CTL services in separate studies and found that a significant majority of users felt helped by either service, with nearly half reporting feeling less suicidal by the end of a crisis chat[31] or text.[32] Interestingly, the digital helplines showed strikingly different user profiles than phone lines, with the most common user for chat and text presenting as young (under 25), female (65% and 79%, respectively), and—in relation to crisis chat services—significantly more likely to be suicidal than callers. For example, CTL users presented with the same frequencies of suicidality as the Lifeline (23%),[32] while Lifeline crisis chat users presented suicidal thoughts or behaviors a remarkable 84% of the time.[31]

988 AND ITS IMPACT ON FUTURE BEHAVIORAL HEALTH SYSTEMS
Federal Action to Implement 988

Recognizing suicide as a major public health priority, Senator Orrin Hatch and Representative Chris Stewart of Utah introduced the National Suicide Hotline Improvement Act of 2018 with near unanimous bipartisan Congressional support. The Act required the FCC to coordinate with SAMHSA and the Department of Veterans Affairs (VA) to study the effectiveness, impact, and feasibility of establishing a 3-digit number for the National Suicide Prevention Lifeline, toward promoting immediate access to suicide prevention and crisis care resources.[33] In 2019, the FCC received reports from SAMHSA and the VA that affirmed the effectiveness of their crisis services and supported the value of assigning an easier to remember and dial 3-digit number to this national hotline network. Citing the known effectiveness of the Lifeline, the FCC subsequently assigned 988 to the Lifeline in July 2020 and Congress authorized the program in The National Suicide Hotline Designation Act in October of the same year.[34,35] The FCC required that the 988 Suicide and Crisis Lifeline be accessible on all telephone platforms across the United States and its territories by July 16, 2022, via phone and text.[34] As indicated in its new name, the Suicide and Crisis Lifeline would also be designed and promoted to address all behavioral health crises (substance use and mental health), in addition to persons in suicidal crisis.

National and State Ramp-Up for 988 Launch

To mobilize and scale behavioral health and crisis systems capacity to successfully launch 988 in July 2022, the executive and legislative branches of federal government, SAMHSA, Vibrant, the Lifeline network centers, and all states (with the help of NASMHPD) would need to work together in ways that were unprecedented. In January 2021, Vibrant provided $10 million in private funds for "988 state planning grants," which were subsequently awarded to the 46 states, Washington D.C., and 3 territories that applied for them.[36] In December 2021, SAMHSA provided $282 million to Vibrant and the states to shore up the 988 crisis network infrastructure. Grants were provided to the states to supplement local funds to enhance local 988 crisis center response, while Vibrant received federal support to expand national back-up center capacity for phones, text, and chat services. Vibrant was also required to apply funds toward enhancing the Lifeline sub-network for Spanish language-speakers and explore pilots for other specialized services [lesbian, gay, bisexual, transgender, queer or questioning, or another diverse gender identity (LGBTQ+) youth, American Indian/Alaskan Natives (AI/AN), and so forth].[37]

Areas of Public Concern and Challenges Related to 988 Implementations

Now that 988 crisis centers were becoming more integrated with the country's behavioral health crisis systems, the very suspicions that spurred their creation in 1960s began to rear their head for some mental health advocates. Would 988 remain anonymous, free, equitable, and be less prone to invasive and coercive practices than the systems they were now integrating with? Some communities expressed worries about 988's potential interface with 911, fearing even more police interventions into mental health crises. These fears, advocates noted, could undermine public trust in 988 and prevent some from calling this more accessible number.[38]

Lifeline's Director noted that callers would continue to be serviced if they wished to remain anonymous, and that policies, practices, and trainings were in place to keep people safe without emergency services intervention in the great majority of contacts. However, there would remain the "last resort" circumstances where emergency service responses would be the only means for keeping 988 callers and related community members safe from imminent harm.[38]

Many of the privacy concerns raised by 988 critics have related to geolocation, that is, a mechanism for potentially giving 988 the same capability as 911 to precisely locate individuals at IR to connect them with emergency services, with or without their consent. As required by Congress, the FCC provided a detailed report on 988 geolocation to explore its cost and feasibility for this service.[39] The report identified "georouting" as a distinct issue for 988, separate from geolocation's fine-tuned tracking capability designed for 911 dispatch. The report noted that Lifeline's centralized routing system has historically routed calls to the nearest local center based on the area code registered to the caller's phone, an unreliable predictor of a caller's location given that most callers are using mobile devices. If the caller *is not* connected to the nearest center, the responder is less able to connect them to local services that could keep them safe and supported after the call, including alternatives to 911 such as mobile crisis or crisis receiving facilities. Consequently, the FCC and SAMHSA are pursuing means of enabling georouting—sending calls to the cell tower nearest the caller—so that callers can receive the benefits of connecting with the centers nearest to them without having their precise location information available to 988 counselors.[39]

The potential interface between 988 and 911 has highlighted both challenges and opportunities for responding to behavioral health crises and emergencies. On one hand, the lack of geolocation capabilities for 988 call, text, or chat users seriously inhibits rapid emergency response for callers at highest risk who are unwilling or unable to inform the counselor where they are.[39] This is particularly noteworthy insofar as 8% of suicide-related calls to the service involve suicides in progress.[15] Consequently, Vibrant and the National Emergency Number Association co-developed an interoperability standard for Lifeline call, text, and chat users to guide 911 operators and 988 counselors on collaborative strategies to respond to users at highest risk whose location was unknown.[40]

Conversely, a significant proportion of 911 callers present with non-emergent behavioral health crises (estimated to be approximately 6%—over 14 million—of 911 callers annually[2]), callers whom could be better served by 988. Several counties around the country have seized upon this opportunity by implementing effective models of diverting non-emergent mental health calls from local public-safety answering points to local 988 centers.[41]

There were also 988 pre-launch concerns related to counselor workforce shortages. Both counselor recruitment and retention issues were reported by 988 crisis centers, with 911 experts raising worries about similar responder burnout problems anticipated for 988 staff. Several centers sought to attract more staff by increasing salaries with increased funding, while SAMHSA established a web site to promote public awareness of 988 counselor job openings at centers.[42]

988 Post-launch and Future Considerations

By July 2022, a crisis hotline number—once seen as an alternative to a traditional mental health service—became a front door to the nation's behavioral health system for all people in crisis. A month after 988's launch, SAMHSA reported that federal and state investments in 988 had significantly improved the overall response rate for the service, citing 152,000 more contacts than the same month a year before, and an overall reduced wait time for all modes of contact from 2.5 minutes to 42 seconds.[43] At that time, SAMHSA began providing network-wide 988 response data to the public on their 988 web site,[44] while Vibrant continued to provide state-level 988 performance metrics on their site.[45]

An independent analysis of Vibrant data by the Kaiser Family Foundation showed that in its first year of service, 988 achieved a 93% overall answer rate by May 2023, a notable improvement over the 70% answer rate reported the same month the year before. As illustrated in **Fig. 2**, this achievement was driven largely by the major federal investments in the nationally centralized chat and text subnetwork response, which was necessary due to sparse local within-state digital crisis care capacity. In its first year, 988 centers (including the VCL) responded to almost 5 million contacts, up 33% from May 2023 compared to May 2022.[46]

With the initial launch successfully completed, SAMHSA received $502 million in fiscal year (FY) 2023 and another $836 million in 2024 to support a variety of national, state, and local 988 crisis care services.[47] For the 988 network, the funding allowed for the realization of long-desired specialized services for underserved and high-risk populations.

- *LGBTQ+ youth ("press 3" option).* In the fall of 2022, Vibrant established a pilot initiative with the Trevor Project to extend help to the high-suicide-risk LGBTQ+ youth population. The phone, text, and chat service grew to 24/7 with a larger subnetwork of centers in 2023, with approximately 1 in every 10,988 (non-Spanish language) users accessing this "press 3" service.[44,48]
- *The capacity for the 988 Spanish-language ("press 2") response was strengthened,* further adding chat and text help for Spanish-speakers in 2023.[49] At the end of 2023, around 1 of every 41 (non-LGBTQ+) 988 users sought assistance in a Spanish language.[44]
- *American Sign Language (ASL) service for deaf and hard of hearing populations.* In the fall of 2023—approximately a year after the groundbreaking 988 LGBTQ + service began—Vibrant rolled out its ASL videophone service ("ASL now" button on 988lifeline.org) for deaf and hard-of-hearing individuals. This service, provided by DeafLEAD, Inc for the SAMHSA-funded Disaster Distress Helpline since 2021, replaced the Lifeline's antiquated and rarely used teletypewriter (TTY) service to extend 24/7 access to 988 through this underserved community's preferred means of communication technology.[50]
- *Washington's Native and Strong Lifeline.* Local legislation enabled 988 AI/AN callers in the state of Washington to attain culturally capable assistance by pressing 4 for the Native and Strong Lifeline in the fall of 2022. This program was the first state-supported helpline program designed to serve the needs of the ethnic group with the highest suicide risk in the country.[51] While this Washington-only program leveraged the national 988 number for access, it broke ground for considering similar state-wide or regional hotline services for AI/AN populations, in line with recommendations made by the US Department of Health and Human Services in 2009.[52]

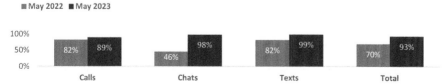

Fig. 2. The Kaiser Family Foundation (KFF) analysis of vibrant emotional health 988 lifeline data, July 14, 2023. (Saunders, H, Taking a Look at 988 Suicide and Crisis Lifeline Implementation One Year After Launch, KFF, July 14,2023. https://www.kff.org/mental-health/issue-brief/taking-a-look-at-988-suicide-crisis-lifeline-implementation-one-year-after-launch/).

988 Transformation of Community Crisis Care Systems

The FY 2023 and 2024 funds previously noted were also intended to support SAMH-SA's vision for extending crisis care well beyond the contact centers responding to calls.[44] SAMHSA expressed a commitment to transform systems to assure that there was "someone to talk to, someone to respond, and a place to go for anyone in crisis, anywhere at any time." As outlined in SAMHSA's National Guidelines for Behavioral Health Crisis Care and their 2021 report to Congress, national, state, and local public health authorities would need to build a full continuum of 24/7 crisis care services, including mobile crisis teams and community crisis receiving facilities. [2,53]

SAMHSA's 5-year vision for 988 began with fortifying funding for the foundation of the service, local member crisis centers. By 2025, SAMHSA aspires for these crisis centers to rapidly facilitate mobile crisis response for at least 80% of the population, with the additional goal of 80% of the country having access to community-based crisis receiving facilities by 2027.[54] In contrasting the role of 988 crisis centers with 911 call centers, SAMHSA noted that crisis hotlines were not in place solely to dispatch and/or connect behavioral health and crisis services with callers; rather, they were themselves an intervention that could resolve crises about 80% of the time.[2]

SUMMARY

For nearly 40 years, crisis and suicide hotlines of the twentieth century were largely viewed as services on the periphery of behavioral health care. Beginning in the twenty-first century, federal funding to network, certify, evaluate, and promote suicide hotlines facilitated greater awareness and credibility for these vital, lifesaving services. The evidence of the National Suicide Prevention Lifeline network's effectiveness was central to the federal government assuring its greater accessibility and visibility in assigning 988 as its new number. In moving from a more peripheral to central position in the nation's behavioral health care system, 988's crisis hotline services will face continuing challenges to meet the evolving needs of both the people seeking help and those seeking to help them. However, 988's transformative potential seems boundless.

As 911 has fueled countless emergency medicine and public safety jobs, intervention tools, and related resources, it is easy to imagine how 988 will do the same for crisis services in America. However, 911's limits in resolving public health and safety emergencies have generated public awareness of the need for earlier prevention approaches, ranging from nutrition education and smoke alarms to defensive driving and self-defense courses. Similarly, this century's 988 service could energize more upstream public mental health education and self-care efforts nationwide. Above all, a fully realized vision of 988 could significantly reduce the stigma, discrimination, and institutionalization of people in mental health crises that resulted from the public safety responses of America's twentieth century.

CLINICS CARE POINTS

- Suicide risk assessments should assess for an individual's desire for suicide (thoughts, etc.), intent for suicide (plans, preparatory behaviors, etc.), capability (past attempts, available means, etc) and buffers against suicide (reasons for living, etc.).

- For effective crisis counseling with individuals in suicidal crisis, establishing good contact (rapport, empathy, etc.) and collaborative problem solving (safety planning, etc.) are essential to good outcomes.

- For persons at imminent risk of suicide, counselors must make every effort to actively engage and collaborate with individuals towards empowering them to secure their own safety, pursuing the least invasive interventions to prevent their suicide.
- In the event an individual is unwilling or unable to collaborate with a counselor to prevent their suicide, and the counselor's assessment of risk indicates the person is likely to seriously harm or kill themselves if they do not act, the counselor must take every reasonable action to prevent their suicide, including contacting emergency response services.
- For persons who state some risk of suicide, counselors should engage them in safety planning and gain consent to pursue follow-up contacts, maintaining engagement with the individual until they are less in distress, less at risk, and/or linked to ongoing clinical care services.

DISCLOSURE

The content, views and opinions of the authors in this manuscript do not necessarily represent the views of Behavioral Health Link, Inc. nor the Substance Abuse and Mental Health Administration or any other branch of the U.S. Government.

REFERENCES

1. Federal Communications Commission, Report on the national suicide hotline improvement act of 2018, 2019, Wireline Competition Bureau; Washington, D.C., Available at: https://docs.fcc.gov/public/attachments/DOC-359095A1.pdf. Accessed February 2, 2024.
2. Substance Abuse and Mental Health Services Administration, 988 Appropriations Report to Congress. 117th Congress, Available at: https://www.samhsa.gov/sites/default/files/988-appropriations-report.pdf, 2021. Accessed February 2, 2024.
3. Sharfstein SS. What ever happened to community mental health? Psychiatr Serv 2000;51(5):616–20.
4. Lamb HR, Weinberger LE, DeCuir WJ Jr. The police and mental health. Psychiatr Serv 2002;53(10):1266–71.
5. Litman RE, Farberow NL, Shneidman ES, et al. Suicide prevention telephone service. JAMA 1965 April 5;192(1):107–11.
6. Brockopp GW. Seven Predictions for SP in the 70's. Crisis Interv 1970;2(1):3.
7. History of the American Association of Suicidology, American Association of Suicidology, Available at: https://suicidology.org/history/. Accessed February 2, 2024.
8. McGee RK, Berg D, Brockopp GW, et al. The Delivery of Crisis Intervention Services. In: Resnik HLP, Hathorne BC, editors. Suicide prevention in the 70's. Rockville, MD: National Institute of Mental Health (U.S.). Center for Studies of Suicide Prevention; 1973. p. 81–90.
9. Technical Assistance Collaborative (TAC). A community-based comprehensive psychiatric crisis response service. Boston, MA: Technical Assistance Collaborative; 2005.
10. Stroul B. Psychiatric crisis response systems: a descriptive study. center for mental health services. SAMHSA 1993.
11. Lester D. The effectiveness of suicide prevention and crisis intervention services. In: Lester D, Rogers J, editors. Crisis intervention and counselling by telephone and the internet. Illinois: Charles C. Thomas; 2012. p. 411–21.
12. Everett A. Groundbreaking Developments in Suicide Prevention and Mental Health Crisis Service Provision, Available at: https://www.samhsa.gov/blog/ground

breaking-developments-suicide-prevention-mental-health-crisis-service-provision, 2021. Accessed February 2, 2024.

13. Substance Abuse and Mental Health Services Administration (SAMHSA). National suicide hotline improvement act: SAMHSA report to the federal communications commission. Rockville, MD: Center for Mental Health Services Suicide Prevention Branch; 2019.

14. Kalafat J, Gould MS, Munfakh JL, et al. An evaluation of crisis hotline outcomes. Part 1: Nonsuicidal crisis callers. Suicide Life-Threatening Behav 2007;37:322–37.

15. Gould MS, Kalafat J, Harrismunfakh JL, et al. An evaluation of crisis hotline outcomes. Part 2: Suicidal callers. Suicide Life-Threatening Behav 2007;37:338–52.

16. Mishara BL, Chagnon F, Daigle M, et al. Comparing models of helper behavior to actual practice in tele- phone crisis intervention: A silent monitoring study of calls to the U.S. 1-800-SUICIDE net- work. Suicide Life-Threatening Behav 2007;37:291–307.

17. Gould MS, Cross W, Pisani AR, et al. Impact of applied suicide intervention skills training on the national suicide prevention lifeline. Suicide Life-Threatening Behav 2013;43:676–91.

18. Joiner T, Kalafat J, Draper J, et al. Establishing standards for the assessment of suicide risk among callers to the National Suicide Prevention Lifeline. Suicide Life-Threatening Behav 2007;37:353–65.

19. Joiner TE. Why people die by suicide. Cambridge, MA: Harvard University Press; 2005.

20. National Suicide Prevention Lifeline. Lifeline Safety Assessment Model. Available at: https://networkresourcecenter.org/display/practiceguide/Safety+Assessment. [Accessed 25 August 2023].

21. Ramchand R, Jaycox L, Ebener P, et al. Characteristics and proximal outcomes of calls made to suicide crisis hotlines in California. Crisis 2017;38(1):26–35.

22. Draper J, Murphy G, Vega E, et al. Helping callers to the national suicide prevention lifeline who are at imminent risk of suicide: The importance of active engagement, active rescue, and collaboration between crisis and emergency services. Suicide Life-Threatening Behav 2014;45:261–70.

23. Vibrant Emotional Health, 988 suicide and crisis lifeline safety policy.published online december 27, 2022, Available at: https://988lifeline.org/wp-content/uploads/2023/02/FINAL_988_Suicide_and_Crisis_Lifeline_Suicide_Safety_Policy_-3.pdf. Accessed February 2, 2024.

24. Gould MS, Lake AM, Munfakh JL, et al. Helping callers to the national suicide prevention lifeline who are at imminent risk of suicide: Evaluation of caller risk profiles and interventions implemented. Suicide Life-Threatening Behav 2016;46(2):172–90.

25. Motto JA, Bostrom AG. A randomized controlled trial of postcrisis suicide prevention. Psychiatr Serv 2001;52:828–33.

26. Carter GL, Clover K, Whyte IM, et al. Postcards from the EDge: 24-month outcomes of a randomised controlled trial for hospital-treated self-poisoning. Br J Psychiatry 2007;191:548–53.

27. Vaiva G, Ducrocq F, Meyer P, et al. Effect of telephone contact on further suicide attempts in patients discharged from an emergency department: Randomised controlled study. Br Med J 2006;332(7552):1241–5.

28. Fleischmann A, Bertolote JM, Wasserman D, et al. Effectiveness of brief intervention and contact for suicide attempters: A randomized controlled trial in five countries. Bull World Health Organ 2008;86:703–9.

29. Gould MS, Lake AM, Galfalvy H, et al. Follow-up with callers to the national suicide prevention lifeline: Evaluation of callers' perceptions of care. Suicide Life-Threatening Behav 2018;48(1):75–86.

30. Britton PC, Karras E, Stecker T, et al. Veterans crisis line call outcomes: distress, suicidal ideation, and suicidal urgency. Am J Prev Med 2022;62(5):745–51.

31. Gould MS, Chowdhury S, Lake AM, et al. National Suicide Prevention Lifeline crisis chat interventions: Evaluation of chatters' perceptions of effectiveness. Suicide Life-Threatening Behav 2021;51:1126–37.

32. Gould MS, Pisani A, Gallo C, et al. Crisis Text Line interventions: Evaluation of texters' perceptions of effectiveness. Suicide Life-Threatening Behav 2022;52:583–95.

33. National suicide hotline improvement act of 2018, pub L No. 115-123, 132 Stat 64, 2018. Summary of H.R. 2345-115th Congress (2017-2018).

34. Federal Communications Commission, Order adopting rules to implement the national suicide hotline improvement act of 2018, fcc 20-100, 35 fcc rcd 6687, july 16, 2020, Available at: https://docs.fcc.gov/public/attachments/FCC-20-100A1_Rcd.pdf, 2020. Accessed February 2, 2024.

35. National Suicide Prevention Hotline Designation Act of 2020, Pub L No. 116-172, 134 Stat 815, 2020.

36. Vibrant Emotional Health, Vibrant emotional health to provide state grants in preparation for future 988 dialing code for the national suicide prevention lifeline; 49 states and u.s. territories to receive grant awards [press release], Available at: https://www.vibrant.org/wp-content/uploads/2021/01/Vibrant-988-Planning-Grant-Announcement.pdf, 2021. Accessed February 2, 2024.

37. Substance Abuse and Mental Health Services Administration, HHS Announces Critical Investments to Implement Upcoming 988 Dialing Code for National Suicide Prevention Lifeline [press release], Available at: https://www.samhsa.gov/newsroom/press-announcements/202112201100, 2021. Accessed February 2, 2024.

38. Pattani A. Social media posts warn people not to call 988. Here's what you need to know, 2022, KFF Health News, Available at: https://www.npr.org/sections/health-shots/2022/08/11/1116769071/social-media-posts-warn-people-not-to-call-988-heres-what-you-need-to-know. Accessed February 2, 2024.

39. Federal Communications Commission, Wireline Competition Bureau. 988 Geolocation Report — National Suicide Hotline Designation Act of 2020 (Document No. 371709A1). 117th Congress, Available at: https://docs.fcc.gov/public/attachments/DOC-371709A1.pdf. Accessed February 2, 2024.

40. National Emergency Number Association, NENA Suicide/Crisis Line Interoperability Standard (NENA-STA-001.2-2022, March 4, 2022), Available at: https://988lifeline.org/wp-content/uploads/2022/04/NENA-Suicide-Crisis-Line-Interoperability-Standard-Published-March-2022.pdf, 2022. Accessed February 2, 2024.

41. National Association of Counties, Shaping Crisis Response Spotlight Series (Pew Technical Report).NACo, Available at: https://www.naco.org/resources/shaping-crisis-response-spotlight-series, 2023. Accessed February 2, 2024.

42. Gorenstein D. and Levi R., Call centers struggling to hire for the new nationwide mental health crisis line. Slate, Available at: https://slate.com/technology/2022/06/988-mental-health-crisis-line-hiring.html, 2022. Accessed February 2, 2024.

43. Substance Abuse and Mental Health Services Administration, HHS Secretary: 988 Transition Moves Us Closer to Better Serving the Crisis Care Needs of People

Across America [press release], Available at: https://www.samhsa.gov/newsroom/press-announcements/20220909, 2022. Accessed February 2, 2024.

44. Substance Abuse and Mental Health Services Administration, 988 lifeline performance metrics. SAMHSA, Available at: https://www.samhsa.gov/find-help/988/performance-metrics. Accessed February 2, 2024.

45. Vibrant Emotional Health, 988 State Based Monthly Reports. 988 Suicide and Crisis Lifeline, Available at: https://988lifeline.org/our-network/. Accessed February 2, 2024.

46. Saunders H. Taking a look at 988 suicide and crisis lifeline implementation one year after launch, 2023, KFF, Available at: https://www.kff.org/mental-health/issue-brief/taking-a-look-at-988-suicide-crisis-lifeline-implementation-one-year-after-launch/. Accessed February 2, 2024.

47. Department of Health and Human Services, Budget in brief, fiscal year 2024, 2023, U.S. HHS, Available at: https://www.hhs.gov/sites/default/files/fy-2024-budget-in-brief.pdf. Accessed February 2, 2024.

48. Livingston K., 988 Suicide Lifeline Expanding LGBTQ services with 24/7 chat and text, 2023, ABC News, Available at: https://abcnews.go.com/Politics/988-suicide-lifeline-expanding-lgbtq-services-247-chat/story?id=97452550. Accessed February 2, 2024.

49. Department of Health and Human Services, 988 Suicide & Crisis Lifeline Adds Spanish Text and Chat Service Ahead of One-Year Anniversary [press release], Available at: https://www.hhs.gov/about/news/2023/07/13/988-suicide-crisis-lifeline-adds-spanish-text-chat-service-ahead-one-year-anniversary.html, 2023. Accessed February 2, 2024.

50. Substance Abuse and Mental Health Services Administration, 988 Suicide & Crisis Lifeline Adds American Sign Language Services for Deaf and Hard of Hearing Callers [press release], Available at: https://www.samhsa.gov/newsroom/press-announcements/20230908/988-suicide-crisis-lifeline-adds-american-sign-language-services-deaf-hard-of-hearing-callers, 2023. Accessed February 2, 2024.

51. Washington State Department of Health, Nation's First Native and Strong Lifeline Launches as Part of 988 [press release], Available at: https://doh.wa.gov/newsroom/nations-first-native-and-strong-lifeline-launches-part-988, 2022, November 17. Accessed February 2, 2024.

52. Office of the Assistant Secretary for Planning and Evaluation, An AI/AN suicide hotline: literature review and discussion with experts, 2009, November 14, U.S. Department of Health and Human Services, Available at: https://aspe.hhs.gov/reports/aian-suicide-prevention-hotline-literature-review-discussion-experts. Accessed February 2, 2024.

53. Substance Abuse and Mental Health Services Administration, National Guidelines for Behavioral Health Crisis Care—A Best Practice Toolkit. Knowledge Informing Transformation, *SAMHSA*, 2020, Available at: https://www.samhsa.gov/sites/default/files/national-guidelines-for-behavioral-health-crisis-care-02242020.pdf. Accessed February 2, 2024.

54. Substance Abuse and Mental Health Services Administration (SAMHSA), Palmieri J. Implementing the SAMHSA and NASMHPD 988 convening playbooks. Washington, D.C: TA Coalition Webinar; 2022.

Community-Based Mental Health Crisis Response

An Overview of Models and Workforce Implications

Michael T. Compton, MD, MPH[a,b,*], Leah G. Pope, PhD[a,b],
Amy C. Watson, PhD[c]

KEYWORDS

- Crisis intervention • Crisis response • Emergency medical services
- Mental health crisis • Mobile crisis • Psychiatric emergency

KEY POINTS

- Improving community-based mental health crisis response is a priority both for the mental health services sector and for law enforcement agencies, with a generally recognized goal of shifting as much of the response as possible away from law enforcement.
- Mobile crisis teams and other multidisciplinary teams are increasingly implemented as part of the service array of local community mental health agencies, though great variations in models exist.
- Among mental health crisis response models embedded within the law enforcement sector, the most widely implemented is Crisis Intervention Team, which provides select officers with specialized training.
- Across all community-based mental health crisis response approaches, workforce implications must be considered both nationally and when local communities choose among models.

INTRODUCTION

In comparison to the general population, individuals with mental illnesses are more likely to have police encounters, more likely to get arrested, more likely to receive a jail sentence for misdemeanors, spend longer in jail, spend longer on probation, and have more probation violations. Those experiencing a mental health crisis are also

[a] Department of Psychiatry, Columbia University Vagelos College of Physicians and Surgeons, New York, NY, USA; [b] New York State Psychiatric Institute, New York, NY, USA; [c] School of Social Work, Wayne State University, Deroit, MI, USA
* Corresponding author. Columbia University Vagelos College of Physicians and Surgeons, 722 West 168th Street, Room R249, New York, NY 10032.
E-mail address: mtc2176@cumc.columbia.edu

Psychiatr Clin N Am 47 (2024) 491–509
https://doi.org/10.1016/j.psc.2024.04.004
0193-953X/24/© 2024 Elsevier Inc. All rights reserved.

likely to have law enforcement responses given the structure of the 911 system and reliance on officers to address disturbances, conflicts, and crises; and they are over-represented among people who are killed by police. Many efforts are underway to decriminalize mental illnesses, with the most promising ones correctly positioned at Intercept 0 (community-based mental health services) and Intercept 1 (emergency call-taking, dispatch, crisis response, and law enforcement) of the Sequential Intercept Model,[1] which details points along the criminal legal system traversed by individuals with mental illnesses and substance use disorders, thus helping communities identify gaps and resources in mental health services at each intercept and develop local action plans. Dissemination of non-law enforcement responders such as a mobile crisis team (MCT) as well as the roll-out of 988 are 2 of the major advances supporting reform and improvement in this area.

Community-based mental health crisis response models, though varying in terms of structure, staffing, and processes, have proliferated across the United States in recent years. Some have been developed in accordance with federal guidelines[2] and/or national expert guidelines,[3] while others have been created or tailored locally to meet a jurisdiction's needs based on contexts such as rurality,[4] the demographics of call subjects such as responses for children and youth,[5] or the specific characteristics of the local mental health system. Law enforcement (eg, municipal police department officers, county sheriff's office deputies, state police) has historically and continues to play a major role in community-based mental health crisis response. This has been driven in part by the use of 911 as the emergency number for both mental health crises and physical health emergencies, the former typically initiating a law enforcement response rather than an emergency medical services response. Reliance on law enforcement for crisis response has also been—and continues to be—underpinned by the very limited existence of non-law enforcement crisis response options. With the introduction of the national 988 number for mental health crises, and the expansion of community-based mental health crisis response models that do not involve law enforcement, the landscape in this area is rapidly evolving. With the possibility of more crisis response options available in any given community (perhaps if only 2 instead of 1), the initiation of one response over the other may hinge on factors such as the caller and the nature of their request for assistance, the number called (eg, 911 vs 988), how the call-taker (and potentially the dispatcher) understands and interprets the caller and the request, and the availability of crisis responders in terms of staffing coverage and availability.

Here, the authors provide an overview of both non-law enforcement-based mental health crisis response models (perhaps best exemplified by MCTs, emergency medical services [EMS]-based, and community responder models) and law enforcement-based mental health crisis response (the most widely known being Crisis Intervention Team [CIT] and co-responder models). Workforce implications are discussed, as are some special considerations with regard to the inclusion of peers with lived experience, race equity, safety concerns, rural versus urban settings, and transportation and involuntary holds.

NON-LAW ENFORCEMENT-BASED RESPONSE MODELS

As noted, community-based mental health crisis response models have proliferated in recent years, with a widely agreed-upon preference for models that do not involve law enforcement. Reasons for this preference include insufficient professional training in this area among officers; crisis response being outside of their crime-fighting and public safety purview; the "criminalization" of mental health conditions by virtue of police presence; elevated risk for misdemeanor charges, arrest, and jail detention (with subsequent criminal justice and mental health sequelae) for behaviors for which other actions would be more appropriate and just; and the risk of using force, resulting in a range of injuries spanning from minor to deadly. Given these concerns, many localities are increasingly shifting toward and investing in non-law enforcement-based response models like mobile crisis and multidisciplinary response teams. On the other hand, some non-law enforcement-based response models have been in existence for decades, such as deploying EMS for some mental health emergencies, but with varying use depending on local contexts. Non-law enforcement-based response models are described below and summarized in **Table 1**.

Mobile Crisis and Multidisciplinary Response Teams

Mobile crisis teams (MCTs) are multidisciplinary response teams composed of some constellation of social workers, nurses, psychiatrists, mental health technicians, and peer specialists. Defined by the Substance Abuse and Mental Health Services Administration (SAMHSA) as a core element of a "no-wrong door, integrated crisis system," MCTs are designed to reach people in their homes, workplaces, or other community-based locations in a timely manner.[2] MCTs have the goal of providing the most effective and least restrictive response for people in mental health crisis with the aim of resolving crises in the community and thereby reducing unnecessary emergency department referrals and hospitalizations.

MCTs have proliferated in the United States since the 1960s, having evolved from earlier psychiatric home-visiting teams and community-based crisis services and today encompassing a wide range of models that vary in staffing, services, target population served, and availability. Teams are generally housed in a community mental health agency or hospital and are dispatched through local crisis lines or community referrals, though police involvement is not uncommon.[6] MCTs must include a licensed and/or credentialed clinician capable of assessing individual needs, but most communities utilize at least 2-person teams that include both professional and paraprofessional staff. For example, many communities now include a peer support worker alongside a bachelor's-level or master's-level clinician; SAMHSA outlines the inclusion of peers within the MCT as a suggestion to fully align with best practice guidelines.

Once on scene, MCTs fulfill a variety of functions, including triage and screening (and explicitly screening for suicidality), assessment, de-escalation, peer support, coordination with medical and behavioral health services, and crisis planning and follow-up.[2] These services can be used to determine the most appropriate response for the person, including facilitating (re)connections to community-based services and resolving the situation to prevent needing a higher level of care. While it is most common for MCTs to serve as a primary response to a crisis call and operate independently of police (and not typically dispatched by the 911 system), it is not uncommon for MCTs to have partnerships with local law enforcement agencies and to provide a secondary response to individuals identified by officers. In Rochester, New York, for example, the Person in Crisis Team was launched in January 2021 by the Rochester Department of Recreation and Human Services; it can be accessed by calling 211 or 988 as well as through 911, and police arriving to a scene can request the team to be called out as well. MCTs may also request law enforcement support when responding to situations in which safety concerns are present.

While much of the literature on MCTs is outdated and lacks methodological rigor, studies have demonstrated that MCT services have high rates of consumer and provider satisfaction, reduce reliance on psychiatric emergency departments, and increase connection to community-based care.[6,7] Commonly cited challenges relate

Table 1 Non-law enforcement-based response models			
	Mobile Crisis Teams		**Emergency Medical Services-Based Teams**	**Other Types of Community Responder Teams**
Who's on the team?	Behavioral health clinician(s)	Behavioral health clinician(s) + peer support worker	Emergency medical technician or paramedic + crisis worker or behavioral health clinician; may include peers	Crisis workers, including peers
Where do calls come from, or how are they dispatched?	Crisis lines, community mental health agencies; sometimes 911		911	Outside agency line (eg, 211, 311, 988), local crisis lines; sometimes 911
Where is the team housed?	Community mental health agency or municipal agency		Municipal agency or other	Municipal agency or other
Examples	Mobile Crisis Response (statewide programs in many states), EMCOT (Austin, TX), PIC Team (Rochester, NY)	MCOT (Salt Lake City, UT), MCRT (San Diego, CA)	Crisis Assistance Helping Out on the Street (CAHOOTS) (Eugene) STAR (Denver, CO), CARE Team (Flagstaff, AZ)	Policing alternatives and diversion (PAD) (Eugene) PAD Initiative (Atlanta, GA), CRU (Olympia, WA)

Abbreviations: CARE, community alliance, response, and engagement; CRU, crisis response unit; EMCOT, expanded mobile crisis outreach team; MCOT, mobile crisis outreach team; MCRT, mobile crisis responder team; PAD, policing alternatives and diversion; PIC, person in crisis; STAR, support team assisted response.

to lengthy response times or limited availability (both in terms of limited operational hours and/or lack of sufficient staffing to meet demand). Given the wide variability in MCT program elements and implementation, additional research is needed regarding effectiveness.

Emergency Medical Services-Based Response

Some communities in the United States and elsewhere are choosing to implement crisis response teams housed within EMS agencies and/or incorporating EMS personnel such as emergency medical technicians (EMTs) or paramedics. The model typically pairs a mental health clinician with the EMS professional, and sometimes a certified peer support worker. Teams are usually, although not exclusively, housed within an EMS agency or fire department, and dispatched via the 911 system. One version of this model is the Psychiatric Ambulance Model (PAM), which has been implemented outside of the United States in countries such as Australia, Sweden, and the Netherlands.[8] PAM teams are typically composed of paramedics and psychiatric nurses who respond to mental health emergency calls in a modified ambulance outfitted with chairs rather than a gurney.

In the past few years, examples of EMS-based responses have also emerged in the United States. This includes the Denver (CO) Support Team Assisted Response

(STAR) program,[9] the Portland (OR) Street Response (PSR),[10] and the Flagstaff (AZ) Community Alliance Response and Engagement (CARE) team.[11] Each of these programs represents collaboration across health and safety agencies, and 2 of the 3 are housed within fire departments responsible for EMS response (PSR and CARE). STAR is managed by the Denver Department of Public Health and Environment in partnership with Denver Public Safety. These programs pair a mental health clinician with an EMT or paramedic to respond to low-risk mental health and behavioral health-related 911 calls for service (eg, welfare checks, suicidal persons, behavioral disturbances). PSR teams also include peer specialists and community health workers who conduct follow-up visits. A significant portion of calls handled by these teams involve people experiencing houselessness and substance intoxication. While these teams may respond at the request of law enforcement, when responding to directly dispatched calls, they rarely, if ever, engage police for support.

Also included in this category are response teams that include a team member with medical training (EMT, nurse), but are not housed within an EMS, fire, or public safety agency. The most well-known example is the Crisis Assistance Helping Out on the Street (CAHOOTS) model developed by and housed within the White Bird Clinic (Eugene, OR), a nonprofit, Federally Qualified Health Center that provides primary medical and behavioral health care. Funded via a contract with the Eugene Police Department, CAHOOTS teams are composed of a crisis worker and a medic (EMT or nurse) and are dispatched by the Eugene emergency communications center to non-violent, mental health-related crises, interpersonal conflicts, welfare checks, substance abuse-related crises, suicidal persons, and non-emergent medical calls. Similar to the EMS-based models housed within EMS agencies, CAHOOTS teams responding to directly dispatched calls rarely need to request law enforcement assistance.

The empirical literature on EMS-based responses is limited. PAM teams outside of the United States have been in operation for over a decade, with some evidence that the PAM response may reduce both police involvement and admission to emergency departments[8,12,13] and is experienced positively by clients.[14] Peer-reviewed research on EMS-based programs in the United States is limited to 1 peer-reviewed article reporting findings from the Denver STAR program. Dee & Pyne[15] examined data from the initial 6-month pilot run of the model. During that period, roughly one-third of Denver STAR calls were at the request of responding police—the remaining two-thirds were directly dispatched to STAR and handled without police involvement, arrest, or injury. Compared to the 6 months prior to STAR implementation, reports of minor crime in the 8 pilot districts decreased by 34%.[15] Evaluation reports (not peer reviewed) on EMS-based programs in the United States suggest that these programs reduce law enforcement involvement. For example, an analysis of the CAHOOTS program data conducted by the Eugene Police Department indicates that 5% to 8% of calls that would have otherwise been handled by police were diverted to CAHOOTS teams,[16] and PSR estimates reducing police response to emergency calls by 3.2% and non-emergency calls by 18.7%.[10] EMS-based teams may also reduce transports to emergency departments[11] and connect clients to clinical and social services.[9]

Other Types of Community Responder Models

In addition to MCTs and EMS-based crisis responses, some communities have opted to design new community responder models that rely on civilians who come from a variety of professional backgrounds. Individuals hired by existing community responder programs include unlicensed behavioral health specialists, community health workers, community members trained in crisis response, harm reduction specialists, and peer support workers, among others. The programs themselves may be operated through existing municipal agencies, through the creation of new agencies, or through existing community-based non-profits. In many cases, these new community responder models have been developed with explicit attention to avoiding police involvement and centering anti-racist and equitable responses, particularly in communities with large Black, Indigenous, and People of Color populations.[17] The Police Alternatives & Diversion (PAD) initiative in Atlanta, Georgia is an example of a community responder model that supports a new approach to civilian response. PAD is an independent non-profit with teams responding to a range of non-crisis situations to address concerns related to extreme poverty, problematic substance use, and mental health. PAD's goal is to reduce arrest and incarceration and increase the availability of and connection to supportive services.

Like the other non-law enforcement-based response models, community responder models are dispatched in a variety of ways across the communities where they are located. PAD, for example, is dispatched through 2 avenues. Community members can call the City of Atlanta's 311 non-emergency services line to make a referral. Alternatively, the Atlanta Police Department or the city's transit police can call the PAD team as an alternative to arrest for individuals detained for law violations related to mental health, substance use, or poverty, who give their consent for a referral. In this case, no police report is made. Given the different avenues through which PAD and other community responder teams may be dispatched to respond to people in need of assistance, communities have developed different strategies for triaging calls and ensuring there is clear guidance on when and how to connect people with the teams. Again, like the other non-law enforcement-based response models, this involves developing protocols for routing calls, including identifying a clear list of call types that are appropriate for community responder teams. Such protocol development often involves collaboration across local public safety and health agencies, which provides opportunities to build trust and collectively decide on which calls are appropriate for referral. In Amherst, Massachusetts, for example, Community Responders for Equity, Safety, and Service (CRESS) was launched in 2022 and can be accessed by the public for low-level calls related to issues concerning mental health, addiction, homelessness, vagrancy, and trespassing. The CRESS team is simultaneously working with its local 911 system to develop protocols for direct dispatch for people who call 911.

The literature on community responder models that do not involve licensed mental health or EMS professionals is limited given that they have only recently been developed. Some internal program evaluations have been completed, however, and new guidance documents offer recommendations for how to effectively capture data across a range of key performance metrics.[18,19]

Workforce Implications for Non-Law Enforcement-Based Models

The expanded investment in non-law enforcement-based models of crisis response raises several implications for the workforce. The authors review 4 key implications here. First, a sustainable workforce for non-law enforcement crisis response does not yet exist and needs to be created. Given the widely recognized behavioral health workforce shortages, there are simply not enough professionals to staff programs throughout the country. For programs that employ licensed mental health professionals, although the Bureau of Labor Statistics estimates that there are enough master's level clinicians to meet demand through 2030, only a small portion of those clinicians are willing to do 24/7 crisis response work in the community.[20] EMS agencies are also struggling to fill positions, reporting fewer candidates for open positions and high rates of turnover (36% for EMTs and 27% for paramedics in 2022).[21] As municipalities struggle to figure out how to best staff new programs with the existing workforce, it has become increasingly clear that new kinds of professionals are needed.

Second, and related to the issue of staffing shortages, a sustainable crisis response workforce depends on building multiple, equitable pathways to becoming a behavioral health crisis responder. This requires focusing on the core skills and capacities that community-based crisis work requires rather than graduate-level or post-graduate-level training and certification that limits entry to the field for many people best-suited for crisis response work.[22]

Third, recruiting crisis responders who reflect the communities they serve and have lived experience will be essential for establishing legitimacy and community buy-in and for promoting equitable responses. The existing behavioral health workforce is disproportionately White, which likely exacerbates racial disparities in mental health service use.[23] The starkest underrepresentation exists with Black and Latinx providers, the same populations overrepresented in the criminal legal system. Increasingly, there is recognition that addressing structural racism in mental health and criminal legal systems requires a diversified workforce.[24] With respect to hiring within non-law enforcement-based models, some communities have expanded their hiring process to recruit more responders of color; other communities have made local residency a requirement for employment to ensure that responders are familiar with and comfortable with the community and its residents.[17] Further, guidance on training for crisis responders often now explicitly includes recommendations to provide training on topics such as anti-racism and anti-oppression, in addition to cultural humility/competency.[25]

Finally, the expansion of non-law enforcement-based models that include several types of professionals brings forward the issue of pay equity in the crisis response field. Staffing shortages in behavioral health have long been linked to historically low wages in the field, which not only lead to difficulties in recruiting qualified providers but also contribute to high burnout and turnover rates.[26] Pay disparities among team members is also an issue as more teams comprise a mix of licensed/unlicensed mental health and civilian responders and evidence suggests that the majority of people of color remain in entry-level and lower paying jobs with little opportunity for advancement.[27] Thus, developing strategies to align compensation for crisis responders with other first responders (eg, law enforcement) and considering issues around equitable pay across roles within a team will be critical for sustaining community-based crisis responder models.

LAW ENFORCEMENT-BASED RESPONSE MODELS

As previously pointed out, mental health crisis response has traditionally relied heavily on the 911 system and the dispatch of law enforcement for behavioral disturbances, complaints with a concern about suspicious persons or behaviors, and even suicidality. Police departments, sheriff's offices, and state police have thus implemented programs to facilitate and improve upon their work in this area. While the Crisis Intervention Team (CIT) model—initially created in 1988 in response to a fatal police shooting of a Black man with a serious mental illness in Memphis, Tennessee—is often considered the premier approach, other models have been developed, typically to complement and augment an agency's CIT program. In addition to crisis response per se, whether dispatched formally (eg, through a 911 public safety answering point) or informally (eg, when an officer asks a CIT-trained officer for assistance), law enforcement officers will continue—even in the context of local implementation of non-law enforcement-based response models like MCTs—to come upon and interact with individuals with mental illnesses (and those in mental health crisis) as part of their routine patrol duties. Additionally, some mental health crisis situations involve significant safety and/or criminal elements; for these reasons, law enforcement will continue to have a role in mental health crisis response, and law enforcement agencies will continue to need to implement programs to enhance their work in the area of mental health crisis response.

Crisis Intervention Team

CIT is a police-based crisis response model implemented in thousands of police departments across the United States, with ongoing dissemination. Specifically, CIT is a community-based collaborative program that has 2 main goals: (1) transforming crisis response systems to minimize the times that law enforcement officers are the first responders to persons with psychiatric disorders or in emotional distress, and (2) ensuring that when officers are first responders, they have the capabilities to de-escalate and divert those experiencing such illnesses or distress from the criminal justice and juvenile justice systems, when possible. The model has garnered broad support from city, county, and state law enforcement agencies. CIT International is a nonprofit membership organization whose purpose is to facilitate understanding, development, and implementation of CIT programs throughout the United States and worldwide. The organization has sponsored annual national conferences over the past 15 years, attracting thousands of law enforcement officers, mental health providers, and advocates. Many state legislatures, state mental health agencies, and state law enforcement training centers support dissemination and implementation of CIT programs. Core Elements of CIT[28] are given in **Box 1**.

One element of a CIT program is CIT training, during which patrol officers receive 40 hours of specialized instruction from police trainers, local mental health professionals, and consumer/family advocates, equipping them with the knowledge, attitudes, and skills to enhance their responses to persons with mental illnesses or those in psychiatric crisis. Although there is some local variation in the week-long curriculum, most curricula include: (1) approximately 14 hours of "didactic" presentations on signs/symptoms, psychotic disorders, mood disorders, personality disorders, substance use disorders, dementia, etc.; (2) about 12 hours of role-play activities in which officers practice verbal and non-verbal de-escalation skills; (3) roughly 6 hours in site visits to local recovery-oriented mental health programs where officers interact with staff, families, and individuals with mental illnesses in recovery and discuss their experiences; (4) about 5 hours of presentations about local community-based mental health services and family/consumer advocacy groups; and (5) several hours set aside for questions/answers and discussion. After training, officers retain their patrol function but become specialized first-line responders when dispatched to mental health calls. In some but not all jurisdictions, emergency call-takers and dispatchers at the local 911 public safety answering point(s) also receive CIT-related training (eg, an abbreviated 8-h version) and thus understand when to specifically dispatch a CIT officer. Controversy exists over the issue of whether CIT should be mandatory for all officers, provided only to self-selected officers who specifically want the training and CIT work, or whether all officers should receive some training with a subset then getting the full CIT training. The Core Elements of the original model suggest that self-selection is important in serving as a CIT officer being dispatched to crisis calls, and that "training all officers" to be CIT officers is not the ideal approach.

Box 1
Core elements of Crisis Intervention Team

Ongoing Elements
1. Partnerships: Law Enforcement, Advocacy, Mental Health
   A. Law Enforcement Community
   B. Advocacy Community
   C. Mental Health Community
2. Community Ownership: Planning, Implementation, & Networking
   A. Planning Groups
   B. Implementation
   C. Networking
3. Policies and Procedures
   A. Crisis Intervention Team (CIT) Training
   B. Law Enforcement Policies and Procedures
   C. Mental Health Emergency Policies and Procedures

Operational Elements
4. CIT: Officer, Dispatcher, Coordinator
   A. CIT Officer
   B. Dispatch
   C. CIT Law Enforcement Coordinator
   D. Mental Health Coordinator
   E. Advocacy Coordinator
   F. Program Coordinator (Multi-jurisdictional)
5. Curriculum: CIT Training
   A. Patrol Officer: 40-Hour Comprehensive Training
   B. Dispatch Training
6. Mental Health Receiving Facility: Emergency Services
   A. Specialized Mental Health Emergency Care

Sustaining Elements
7. Evaluation and Research
   A. Program Evaluation Issues
   B. Development Research Issues
8. In-Service Training
   A. Extended and Advanced Training
9. Recognition and Honors
   A. Examples
10. Outreach: Developing CIT in Other Communities
    A. Outreach Efforts

Relatively extensive descriptive, non-experimental, and quasi-experimental studies have documented that CIT increases the use of mental health service linkages to resolve mental health-related encounters.[29–33] Additionally, CIT can be considered an evidence-based practice in terms of changing officers' knowledge and attitudes.[34,35] The National Institute of Mental Health (NIMH) has funded 2 large quasi-experimental studies—in 6 law enforcement agencies in Georgia and in Chicago, respectively—with consistently positive results,[31,33,36,37] and a NIMH-funded multi-site randomized, controlled trial of CIT training is currently underway (ClinicalTrials. Gov NCT 05606289).

Co-responder Model

The co-responder model (**Table 2**) typically pairs a mental health clinician with a specially trained police officer to respond to mental health crisis calls. Like EMS-

Table 2
Co-responder models

Examples	Primary or Secondary Response	How They Arrive	Team Composition
City of Chicago CARE Team	Primary	Ride together	Officer, clinician, paramedic
Los Angeles Police Department Systemwide Mental Assessment Response Team	Secondary	Ride together	Officer, licensed clinician
Springfield, MO Police Department Virtual-Mobile Crisis Intervention	Officer primary, clinician secondary	Separately, officer with iPad	Officer, licensed clinician
Waukesha County Sheriff's Department	Officer primary, clinician secondary	Separately	Officer, licensed clinician

based models, co-responder models were initially more common outside of the United States. However, this model is rapidly gaining popularity in the United States.[38] Co-responder teams may be implemented as a standalone crisis response approach, or integrated into more comprehensive mental health and policing collaboration efforts that may also include a CIT program and various diversion strategies. Co-responder team programs are designed to divert people with mental illnesses away from the criminal legal system and reduce the need for emergency department transports and hospitalization by providing crisis assessment, stabilization, and connection to services in the community. In the wake of the murder of George Floyd, co-responder teams are also being implemented in attempt to reduce reliance on police in responding to non-criminal events.

Reviews of the literature on the co-responder model suggest significant variation in terms of how teams operate.[39] This variation reflects the tailoring of programs to specific community needs and preferences, as well as available funding, staff, equipment, and behavioral health services. In some communities, such as Los Angeles (CA) and Tucson (AZ), the officer and clinician ride together in a patrol car; in others, such as the Waukesha County (WI) Sheriff's Department, they ride separately; and in still others, such as the Springfield, Missouri Police Department, the officer responds to the scene and the clinician provides remote support via phone or an iPad.[7] There is also variation in terms of when co-responder teams respond. In communities like Tucson, the team is directly dispatched to "hot calls" as the first response; in others, they provide secondary response at the request of a patrol officer, such as Los Angeles Police Department's Systemwide Mental Assessment Response Teams (SMART); and in others, such as the Poulsbo, Washington Police Department, they primarily conduct follow-up visits after a police response.[7,40] While in many communities, co-responder teams are composed of an officer and a licensed clinician, cities such as Chicago (IL) and Dallas (TX), are implementing teams that also include a paramedic.[41,42] Resource options vary by community; thus, co-responder teams may or may not have access to crisis stabilization centers, sobering centers, housing resources, living room models, and peer support services. Other types of program variations pertain to the training of team members, hours of operation, geographic area serviced, and whether officers are in uniform or in plain clothes. Additionally, it should be noted that local models evolve over time as the crisis system matures, and to meet changing local needs. Co-responder models are very popular, though in some jurisdictions, they are just starting points for what will become a more mature system with better triaging and more options based on that triaging. For example, in Tucson, programs have evolved such that officers and clinicians no longer ride together because they found it ineffi-cient across broad geographic areas, and because the officer was often waiting for the clinician to complete their documentation and vice versa. They also tend to no longer respond to most "hot calls" (which might best be handled with a CIT officer or with a MCT response), and now focus more on follow-up and outreach, as a form of "collaborative response."

Research to date indicates some promising outcomes associated with co-responder teams. There is evidence that the model may reduce unnecessary emer-gency department transports and increase service use following the initial contact, reduce short-term incarceration risk, and reduce use of force in situations involving suicidal persons.[39,43–45] There is also evidence that stakeholders find the co-responder model acceptable and many people with mental illnesses and their family members find having a clinician present preferable to police-only response.[46–48]

Other Law Enforcement-Based Models

Although not widespread and with little research or even descriptive literature, other law enforcement-based approaches and models exist. Some law enforcement agencies have created their own "case management" approaches to engagement and follow-up after crisis response or repeated encounters. Such case management service programs, sometimes implemented in collaboration with behavioral health ser-vice providers, are designed to enhance proactive engagement with and response to individuals with serious mental illnesses or other significant health and social service needs.[49] Programs that have been described, despite virtually no research on the approach, include the Houston (TX) Chronic Consumer Stabilization Initiative and the Los Angeles (CA) Police Department's Case Assessment and Management Pro-gram.[49] Both short-term and longer-term individualized response plans are designed to ensure that clients have access to and are connecting with available behavioral health treatment and social services in an effort to reduce repeated contacts with law enforcement personnel.

Other agencies have implemented approaches to directly connect with mental health professionals without fully embedding a clinician with an officer in the way that the co-responder model does. For example, a mental health clinician might be based at a 911 call center or a precinct in order to provide call-takers, dispatchers, or patrol officers with ready access to informal consultation. Other jurisdictions have piloted telepsychiatry-like programs to connect law enforcement officers in the field with mental health professionals using mobile technologies. In another instance, offi-cers access the advice of a mental health clinician through brief telephonic support triggered by a notification system to responding officers.[31,36] The Smart911 system allows someone to create a "safety profile" that includes medical information and lists prescribed medications that, in the event of an emergency call, displays to 911 personnel. Some law enforcement agencies create their own records system so that officers can be alerted if an individual is known to have a mental illness and repeated contacts.

Workforce Implications of Law Enforcement-Based Response Models

With regard to CIT, one of the chief workforce-related challenges centers around the need to pull officers off routine duties for the 5 days of the training, which may be especially problematic for small agencies. Other issues pertain to overtime pay (either for the officers receiving the training or for those covering patrol duties for them) and union-related concerns (eg, in terms of who gets selected for the training). More overarchingly, a workforce challenge for law enforcement agency leadership is having an adequate number of patrol officers trained in order to ensure that CIT-trained officers are available at all times, in keeping with the Core Elements. It has been suggested that to achieve this, 20% to 25% of the agency's patrol division should be trained, especially those self-selecting into the CIT role, though differences exist between large, urban communities and small, rural ones with regard to the ideal percentage. Turnover (eg, retirements, new recruits, and patrol officers advancing to non-patrol positions) must be considered in maintaining an agency's optimal coverage. Similar considerations are true for dispatchers, who benefit from an abbreviated CIT training in order to appropriately elicit sufficient information to identify a mental health-related crisis and dispatch a CIT officer.

In terms of the co-responder model, a key workforce challenge of embedding a mental health clinician with an officer is potential under-utilization of the clinician on calls for which their involvement is actually unnecessary, even if initially (eg, at the time of dispatch) seeming appropriate. Additionally, given that most clinicians' salaries are supported through billing (with billing being unavailable in this context), either the law enforcement agency or the local mental health agency typically has to fund the position. It should be noted, however, that issues pertaining to billing may become less of a barrier as states are building crisis systems using variations in funding streams such as Medicaid Section 1915(c) home and community-based services waivers and Section 1915(i) state plan amendments, as well as certified community behavioral health clinics. Another workforce challenge occurs in agencies with co-response teams in which the officer and clinician ride together. Current patrol unit staffing shortages may be exacerbated when the co-response officer is not available to respond to regular patrol calls.

SPECIAL CONSIDERATIONS

1. *Involving peer support workers.* Peer support workers, or individuals with lived experience, can promote shared understanding and positive coping strategies, while providing information and local resources, across the array of mental health settings. Some of the models described now incorporate peer support workers into the staffing structure of crisis response services. Having a peer support worker—on, for example, an MCT—provides opportunities for individuals in crisis to talk with someone who has had similar experiences, embodies recovery, and offers messages of encouragement and hope.[50] Peer support workers can help in building a trusting relationship, offering calming during a stressful situation, overcoming feelings of isolation and fear, and demonstrating the possibility of recovery. While the benefits are widely recognized, potential challenges to be considered include those related to workforce insufficiency, role integrity, the potential for stigma and discrimination from co-workers, the need to support sustainable employment and fair pay despite not being a licensed mental health professional, and the need to engage in self-care to maintain personal well-being and reduce the risk of burnout or symptom recurrence.[50]

2. *Intentionally addressing race equity.* Given the widely recognized unjust over-representation of people of color in the criminal legal system, as well as inequities in mental health care spanning from diagnosis to treatment outcomes across the array of mental health settings, an intentional focus on race equity is crucial. An antiracist approach—including education and training as well as program development and policy—is needed in efforts to decriminalize mental illnesses, including acute exacerbations and psychiatric crises. One step is to reduce reliance on law enforcement (including the use of 911) to the largest extent possible for mental health crisis response. Diversion to mental health providers and services, however, is not sufficient given known racial inequities and structural harms within the mental health system itself in terms of access, engagement, coercive practices, and provision of evidence-based services.[51] Another strategy pertains to efforts to diversify the mental health workforce, broadly but also in the realm of community-based crisis response. Program planners should commit to using an equity framework in both the design and evaluation of crisis response systems, which includes engaging communities directly in a meaningful and ongoing manner.[51] Without these and other efforts, it is likely that crisis response services will perpetuate rather than minimize racial inequities.

3. *Dissecting "safety concerns" that elicit law enforcement responses.* One set of conscious and unconscious concerns that could impede progress in advancing non-law enforcement crisis response are those about "safety" during such responses. Some mental health services providers, for example, are on the one hand engaged in 988 implementation and MCT expansion, while on the other noting that they would not want to send out the team without police presence, due to "safety concerns." Equally, some law enforcement agencies, despite acknowledging that mental health crisis response is outside of their professional purview, also feel that police presence is necessary, for safety. Safety is indeed a legitimate concern for some crisis response situations, but likely a vague, poorly specified concern (related to fear or liability concerns) for many other types of crisis response situations for which there is little safety risk. Vague "safety concerns" also may represent significant racial bias and may reflect unfounded fears of deploying non-law enforcement-based responses in communities historically viewed as unsafe. If not clearly defined and operationalized, concerns about safety could impede efforts to develop alternative responses and could perpetuate racial inequities in policing and in mental health services delivery.

4. *Considering urban versus rural differences.* The approaches and models described here were developed for and primarily implemented in urban, and perhaps suburban, settings. Several factors complicate implementation in rural (and even more so, remote and frontier) jurisdictions. One pertains to travel distances, and thus promptness of response. Relatedly, low population densities mean that crises are not only geographically dispersed over wide distances, but also rarer, which has implications for staffing and sustainability. Gaps in mental health and social services may also make effective crisis response less attainable. Some solutions include building partnerships between neighboring towns and counties, private service agencies with large service areas, and others; leveraging telehealth technology to shift some service provision to virtual delivery; and, where demand may not be high enough to justify program costs, drawing on existing local resources to develop services tailored to the community's needs.[4]

5. *Determining most appropriate approaches to transportation and involuntary holds.* Although others could be enumerated, a fifth special consideration pertains to transportation, both voluntary and involuntary. Many law enforcement

agencies perceive the mental health system as relying too heavily on them for transportation (eg, to a psychiatric emergency receiving facility, or between psychiatric facilities). Additionally, research and development are needed in the area of identifying the ideal approaches to transport since neither ambulances nor officers' patrol cars are designed to be appropriate for mental health crisis response, or for transport of individuals in mental health crisis. Relatedly, issues around who can, should, or must initiate involuntary holds—and thus involuntary transportation to receiving facilities—would benefit from further cross-disciplinary program and policy deliberations, including policy deliberations at the level of state law.

DISCUSSION: HOW COMMUNITIES CHOOSE AMONG MODELS

Models of community-based mental health crisis response have multiplied over the past decade in an attempt to address the clear shortcomings of a patchwork crisis care system, including unnecessary emergency department use and hospital admissions, overuse of law enforcement, and fatal police encounters that involve people with mental illnesses. In 2020, SAMHSA published national guidelines for crisis care that articulate a coordinated, comprehensive crisis response system as one that includes "someone to talk to" (eg, crisis call centers and 988), "someone to respond" (eg, MCTs), and "a place to go" (eg, crisis receiving and stabilization services).[2] The clear focus on ensuring mobile crisis services that offer community-based intervention to individuals in crisis highlights a need for communities to articulate what their current network of crisis response services looks like and what they ideally would like it to look like. How should communities decide what models—or mix of models—they need?

Available guidance suggests that communities adopt the model(s) that are most appropriate to address community needs. Since the models described earlier are not mutually exclusive, this often means that communities implement multiple response models to create a layered approach to crisis response. The first step in determining what model(s) to implement is to conduct a needs assessment that identifies local needs, existing service gaps, and community assets. Such needs assessments ideally engage a range of stakeholders (eg, law enforcement, 911 call centers, EMS, MCTs, people with direct experience receiving crisis services, family members, advocates) who can collaborate over a specified planning period to identify challenges and potential solutions for their crisis system.[19] This process can result in a clearer articulation of what models are needed in the community and how they can work together to address needs in a sustainable way. This can in turn lead to more concrete planning about what models will be implemented, where they will be located (ie, within what local agency or provider organization), and how they will be staffed.

A second step in determining what model(s) to implement in a community is to consider the relationships that will exist across law enforcement and non-law enforcement-based responders. As the description of models given earlier makes clear, models have varying levels of interaction with the 911 emergency response system and law enforcement agencies. Some models are embedded within a police department and can be dispatched directly from 911 (with or without police as co-responders) while other models exist entirely outside of law enforcement or receive the majority of calls from service providers and community members who do not want to call 911. Even programs that operate separately from police, however, are likely to need some relationship with the police—such as when they need support for situations that escalate or are more dangerous than they first appeared. For this reason, many communities that have implemented non-law enforcement-based response models describe ongoing collaboration with law enforcement in order to get the right resources to the right place at the right time.[52]

Finally, as communities make decisions about what field-based crisis response models to implement, there must be a simultaneous commitment to ongoing data collection and analysis that helps stakeholders understand whether programs are meeting their intended goals and what changes may need to be made. This involves deciding on what metrics are possible to collect and what values of those metrics would indicate program success, who is responsible for collecting data and sharing data across agencies, and partnering with outside organizations that can conduct external evaluations assessing feasibility, acceptability, and outcomes at the individual level, program level, and system level.[19] Because of the variety of models that exist and the various ways in which they are staffed, resourced, and made accessible to the community, it is difficult to compare models and there is currently no standardized way to determine the best model.[53] Given that communities are dynamic ecosystems, they will likely need to continuously monitor the mix of crisis response models in their jurisdictions to ensure that they are continuing to best meet the needs of the population they are intended to serve.

SUMMARY

Wide variation exists in jurisdictions across the United States in terms of the staffing, structure, and approaches of both non-law enforcement-based and law enforcement-based mental health crisis response. Research—on process metrics and on outcomes including client disposition and satisfaction—is generally lacking or outpaced by program implementation. As local communities determine and implement the ideal community-based mental health crisis response models, all approaches should strive to reduce criminal legal system involvement and ensure race equity. Multiple workforce implications and challenges will need to be addressed as models expand and improve.

CLINICS CARE POINTS

- Individuals with behavioral health disorders and serious mental illnesses in particular, are at increased risk for mental health crisis events that are often responded to by law enforcement, which thus increases risk for arrest and further criminal legal system involvement.

- To reduce reliance on law enforcement-based crisis response, efforts are increasingly underway, especially in the era of 988, to enhance and expand non-law enforcement responses, as exemplified by mobile crisis teams.

- Across mental health crisis response approaches—both those that are law enforcement-based and those that are not—workforce implications must be addressed, including, for example, equitable pay.

- As service agencies and local communities plan and evaluate mental health crisis response approaches and models, they should consider involving peer support workers, intentionally address race equity, dissect any safety concerns that might elicit law enforcement responses, consider implications for urban versus rural communities, and determine the most appropriate approaches to transportation and involuntary holds.

DISCLOSURE

The authors report no financial conflicts of interest.

REFERENCES

1. Munetz MR, Griffin PA. Use of the Sequential Intercept Model as an approach to decriminalization of people with serious mental illness. Psychiatr Serv 2006;57(4): 544–9.

2. National Guidelines for Behavioral Health Crisis Care: Best Practice Toolkit. Substance Abuse and Mental Health Services Administration. 2020. Available at: https://www.samhsa.gov/sites/default/files/national-guidelines-for-behavioral-health-crisis-care-02242020.pdf. [Accessed 14 July 2023].

3. Pinals DA. Crisis Services: Meeting Needs, Saving Lives. National Association of State Mental Health Program Directors. Available at: https://store.samhsa.gov/sites/default/files/pep20-08-01-001.pdf. [Accessed 23 June 2023].

4. Tailoring Crisis Response and Pre-Arrest Diversion Models for Rural Communities. Substance Abuse and Mental Health Services Administration. 2019. Available at: https://store.samhsa.gov/product/Tailoring-Crisis-Response-and-Pre-Arrest-Diversion-Models-for-Rural-Communities/PEP19-CRISIS-RURAL. [Accessed 14 July 2023].

5. National Guidelines for Child and Youth Behavioral Health Crisis Care. Substance Abuse and Mental Health Services Administration. 2022. Available at: https://store.samhsa.gov/sites/default/files/SAMHSA_Digital_Download/pep-22-01-02-001.pdf. [Accessed 14 July 2023].

6. Watson AC, Compton MT, Pope LG. Crisis Response Services for People with Mental Illnesses or Intellectual and Developmental Disabilities: A Review of the Literature on Police-based and Other First Response Models. Vera Institute of Justice. 2019. Available at: https://www.vera.org/downloads/publications/crisis-response-services-for-people-with-mental-illnesses-or-intellectual-and-developmental-disabilities.pdf. [Accessed 15 May 2024].

7. Assessing the Impact of Co-Responder Team Programs: A Review of Research. Academic Training to Inform Police Responses: Best Practice Guide. International Association of Chiefs of Police and University of Cincinnati Center for Police Research and Policy. Available at: https://www.theiacp.org/sites/default/files/IDD/Review%20of%20Co-Responder%20Team%20Evaluations.pdf. [Accessed 15 May 2024].

8. De Jong IC, Van der Ham LAJ, Waltz MM. Responding to persons in mental health crisis: A cross-country comparative study of professionals' perspectives on psychiatric ambulance and street triage models. J Community Saf Well Being 2022;7(Suppl_1):S36–44.

9. Denver Public Safety. Support Team Assisted Response (STAR) 2022 Mid-Year Report. Available at: https://www.denvergov.org/files/assets/public/public-health-and-environment/documents/cbh/2022_midyear_starreport_accessible.pdf. [Accessed 27 June 2023].

10. Townley G, Leickly E. Portland Street Response: Year Two Program Evaluation. Portland State University Homelessness Research & Action Collaborative. 2023. Available at: https://www.pdx.edu/homelessness/sites/homelessness.web.wdt.pdx.edu/files/2023-07/HRAC%20Portland%20Street%20Response%20Year%20Two%20Evaluation%20Report_FINAL%20FOR%20WEBSITE.pdf. [Accessed 15 May 2024].

11. Flagstaff Fire Department. January–December 2022 Annual Report. Available at: https://www.flagstaff.az.gov/DocumentCenter/View/76798/2022-Flagstaff-Fire-Department-Annual-Report-Slides-only-?bidId=. [Accessed 27 June 2023].

12. Bouveng O, Bengtsson FA, Carlborg A. First-year follow-up of the Psychiatric Emergency Response Team (PAM) in Stockholm County, Sweden: A descriptive study. Int J Ment Health 2017;46(2):65–73.
13. Kuiper AV. Psychiatric ambulance service for people with a mental illness. Erasmus University Thesis Repository. Available at: http://hdl.handle.net/2105/21880. [Accessed 17 July 2023].
14. Lindström V, Sturesson L, Carlborg A. Patients' experiences of the caring encounter with the psychiatric emergency response team in the emergency medical service—A qualitative interview study. Health Expectations 2020;23(2):442–9.
15. Dee TS, Pyne J. A community response approach to mental health and substance abuse crises reduced crime. Science Advances 2022;8(23). https://doi.org/10.1126/sciadv.abm2106.
16. Eugene Police Department Crime Analysis Unit. CAHOOTS Program Analysis. 2020. Available at: https://www.eugene-or.gov/DocumentCenter/View/56717/CAHOOTS-Program-Analysis. [Accessed 17 July 2023].
17. Beck J, Stagoff-Belfort A, Tan de Bibiana J. Civilian crisis response: a toolkit for equitable alternatives to police response. Vera Institute of Justice; 2022. Available at: https://www.vera.org/civilian-crisis-response-toolkit. [Accessed 28 June 2023].
18. Beck J, Reuland M, Pope L. Behavioral health crisis alternatives: shifting from police to community responses. Vera Institute of Justice; 2020. Available at: https://www.vera.org/behavioral-health-crisis-alternatives. [Accessed 28 June 2023].
19. Council of State Governments Justice Center. Expanding first response: a toolkit for community responder programs. 2021. Available at: https://csgjusticecenter.org/publications/expanding-first-response/. [Accessed 28 June 2023].
20. Bureau of Labor Statistics, U.S. Department of Labor. Occupational outlook handbook, EMTs and paramedics. Available at: https://www.bls.gov/ooh/healthcare/emts-and-paramedics.htm. [Accessed 30 May 2023].
21. NAEMT 2022 National Report on Engagement and Satisfaction in EMS. National Association of Emergency Medical Technicians. 2022. Available at: https://ambulance.org/2022/10/17/4th-annual-study-shows-worsening-ems-turnover/NAEMT. [Accessed 15 May 2024].
22. Carroll JJ, El-Sabawi T, Fichter D, Pope LG, Rafla-Yuan E, Compton MT, Watson A. The workforce for non-police behavioral health crisis response doesn't exist—We need to create it. Health Affairs Blog 2021. Available at: https://ramaonhealthcare.com/the-workforce-for-non-police-behavioral-health-crisis-response-doesnt-exist-we-need-to-create-it/. [Accessed 15 May 2024].
23. Racial/Ethnic Differences in Mental Health Service Use among Adults. Substance Abuse and Mental Health Services Administration. 2015. Available at: https://www.samhsa.gov/data/sites/default/files/MHServicesUseAmongAdults/MHServicesUseAmongAdults.pdf. [Accessed 14 July 2023].
24. Vinson SY, Dennis AL. Systemic, racial justice–informed solutions to shift "care" from the criminal legal system to the mental health care system. Psychiatr Serv 2021;72(12):1428–33.
25. Report on International Crisis Response Team Trainings. Reach Out Response Network. 2021. Available at: https://static1.squarespace.com/static/5f29-dc87171bd201ef5cf275/t/61001cc7a1cba525808a68ee/1627397322046/RORN+Trainings+Report+-+July+27+Final.pdf. [Accessed 14 July 2023].
26. Behavioral Health + Economics Network. Addressing the Behavioral Health Workforce Shortage. Available at: https://www.bhecon.org/wp-content/uploads/2016/

09/BHECON-Behavioral-Health-Workforce-Fact-Sheet-2018.pdf. [Accessed 28 June 2023].

27. State Strategies to Increase Diversity in the Behavioral Health Workforce. National Academy for State Health Policy. 2021. Available at: https://nashp.org/state-strategies-to-increase-diversity-in-the-behavioral-health-workforce/. [Accessed 14 July 2023].

28. Crisis Intervention Team (CIT) Methods for Using Data to Inform Practice: A Step-by-Step Guide. Substance Abuse and Mental Health Services Administration. 2018. Available at: https://store.samhsa.gov/sites/default/files/d7/priv/sma18-5065.pdf. [Accessed 14 July 2023].

29. Teller JLS, Munetz MR, Gil KM, Ritter C. Crisis Intervention Team training for police officers responding to mental disturbance calls. Psychiatr Serv 2006;57(2): 232–7.

30. Watson AC, Ottati VC, Draine J, Morabito M. CIT in context: The impact of mental health resource availability and district saturation on call dispositions. Int J Law Psychiatr 2011;34(4):287–94.

31. Compton MT, Bakeman R, Broussard B, et al. The police-based Crisis Intervention Team (CIT) model: II. Effects on level of force and resolution, referral, and arrest. Psychiatr Serv 2014;65:523–9.

32. Kubiak S, Comartin E, Milanovic E, et al. Countywide implementation of Crisis Intervention Teams: Multiple methods, measures and sustained outcomes. Behav Sci Law 2017;35(5–6):456–69.

33. Watson AC, Owens LK, Wood J, Compton MT. The impact of Crisis Intervention Team response, dispatch coding, and location on the outcomes of police encounters with individuals with mental illnesses in Chicago. Policing (Oxf) 2021; 15(3):1948–62.

34. Compton MT, Bahora M, Watson AC, Oliva JR. A comprehensive review of extant research on Crisis Intervention Team (CIT) programs. J Am Acad Psychiatry Law 2008;36:47–55.

35. Watson AC, Compton MT, Draine JN. The Crisis Intervention Team (CIT) model: An evidence-based policing practice? Behav Sci Law 2017;35(5–6):431–41.

36. Compton MT, Bakeman R, Broussard B, et al. The police-based Crisis Intervention team (CIT) model: I. Effects on officers' knowledge, attitudes, and skills. Psychiatr Serv 2014;65:517–22.

37. Watson AC, Wood JD. Everyday police work during mental health encounters: A study of call resolutions in Chicago and their implications for diversion. Behav Sci Law 2017;35(5–6):442–55.

38. Marcus N, Stergiopoulos V. Re-examining mental health crisis intervention: A rapid review comparing outcomes across police, co-responder and non-police models. Health Soc Care Community 2022;30(5):1665–79.

39. Puntis S, Perfect D, Kirubarajan A, et al. A systematic review of co-responder models of police mental health 'street' triage. BMC Psychiatry 2018;18(1):256. https://doi.org/10.1186/s12888-018-1836-2.

40. Dempsey C, Quanbeck C, Bush C, Kruger K. Decriminalizing mental illness: Specialized policing responses. CNS Spectrums 2020;25(2):181–95.

41. City of Chicago. Crisis Assistance Response and Engagement Program (CARE) Annual Report. Available at: https://www.chicago.gov/content/dam/city/sites/public-safety-and-violenc-reduction/pdfs/CARE%202022-Annual%20Report-12-7.pdf. [Accessed 28 June 2023].

42. Multi-Disciplinary Response Teams. Transforming Emergency Mental Health Response in Texas. Meadows Mental Health Policy Institute; 2021. Available at:

https://mmhpi.org/wp-content/uploads/2021/06/MDRT-Transforming-Crisis-Response-in-Texas.pdf. [Accessed 14 July 2023].

43. Bailey K, Lowder EM, Grommon E, Rising S, Ray BR. Evaluation of a police–mental health co-response team relative to traditional police response in Indianapolis. Psychiatr Serv 2022;73(4):366–73.

44. Blais E, Brisebois D. Improving police responses to suicide-related emergencies: New evidence on the effectiveness of co-response police-mental health programs. Suicide Life Threat Behav 2021;51(6):1095–105.

45. Shapiro GK, Cusi A, Kirst M, O'Campo P, Nakhost A, Stergiopoulos V. Co-responding police-mental health programs: A review. Admin Policy Ment Health 2014;42(5):606–20.

46. Boscarato K, Lee S, Kroschel J, Hollander Y, Brennan A, Warren N. Consumer experience of formal crisis-response services and preferred methods of crisis intervention. Int J Ment Health Nurs 2014;23(4):287–95.

47. Lamanna D, Shapiro GK, Kirst M, Matheson FI, Nakhost A, Stergiopoulos V. Co-responding police-mental health programmes: Service user experiences and outcomes in a large urban centre. Int J Ment Health Nurs 2018;27(2):891–900.

48. Pope LG, Patel A, Fu E, et al. Crisis response model preferences of mental health care clients with prior misdemeanor arrests and of their family and friends. Psychiatr Serv 2023;74(11):1163–70.

49. Law Enforcement-Based Case Management Services: A Review of Research. International Association of Chiefs of Police and University of Cincinnati Center for Police Research and Policy. Available at: https://www.theiacp.org/sites/default/files/IDD/Review%20of%20LE%20Case%20Management%20Services.pdf. [Accessed 14 July 2023].

50. Peer Support Services in Crisis Care. Substance Abuse and Mental Health Services Administration. 2022. Available at: https://store.samhsa.gov/sites/default/files/pep22-06-04-001.pdf. [Accessed 14 July 2023].

51. Goldman ML, Vinson SY. Centering equity in mental health crisis services. World Psychiatry 2022;21(2):243–4.

52. Irwin A, Pearl B. The Community Responder Model: How Cities Can Send the Right Responder to Every 911 Call. Center for American Process. 2020. Available at: https://www.americanprogress.org/article/community-responder-model/. [Accessed 14 July 2023].

53. Curry J, Sloan L, Rush WK, Gulrajani C. The changing landscape of mental health crisis response in the United States. J Am Acad Psychiatr Law 2023;51:6–12.

Crisis Receiving and Stabilization Facilities
Designing Systems for High-Acuity Populations

Margaret E. Balfour, MD, PhD[a,b,*], Chris A. Carson, MD, MBA[c]

KEYWORDS

- Mental health services • Emergency care • Emergency psychiatric services
- Crisis intervention • Health care systems

KEY POINTS

- Crisis facilities provide a safe and therapeutic alternative to jails and emergency departments, but programs vary widely in scope, capability, and populations served.
- Crisis program design should center around the needs of its customers, which include individuals and families in crisis and key community stakeholders such as first responders.
- High-acuity programs include receiving facilities that can quickly accept first-responder drop-offs with a "no wrong door" policy of never turning anyone away and specialized units that provide treatment in a safe and therapeutic environment.
- Lower acuity programs provide a supportive, home-like environment with less medical and nursing involvement for populations that are non-violent and able to engage in care voluntarily.
- Ideally, a crisis system should be organized into a broad continuum of services that ensures care is provided in the least restrictive setting, even for people with high acuity needs, and stakeholders should have a clear understanding of the capabilities of each component facility and the population it can safely serve.

INTRODUCTION

Crisis facilities provide safe and therapeutic alternatives to hospital emergency departments (EDs), inpatient psychiatric units, and jails, and form the third pillar of the Substance Abuse and Mental Health Service Administration vision for behavioral health crisis systems in which everyone has someone to call (the 988 Suicide and Crisis Lifeline), someone to respond (mobile crisis teams), and a safe place for help (specialized crisis facilities).[1] As interest in and financing for crisis services continue

[a] Connections Health Solutions, 2802 East District Street, Tucson, AZ 85714, USA; [b] Department of Psychiatry, University of Arizona College of Medicine, Tucson, AZ, USA; [c] Connections Health Solutions, 2390 East Camelback Road Suite 400, Phoenix, AZ 85016, USA
* Corresponding author.
E-mail address: margie.balfour@connectionshs.org

Psychiatr Clin N Am 47 (2024) 511–530
https://doi.org/10.1016/j.psc.2024.04.022   **psych.theclinics.com**

to grow, communities across the United States are in various stages of planning and building new crisis facilities, with states reporting a more than doubling in the number of facilities from 2022 to 2023.[2] This expansion creates an unprecedented opportunity to build and organize systems that ensure all populations are served in the least restrictive setting that safely meets their needs.

However, the landscape of crisis facilities can be complex and confusing. Crisis facilities vary widely in scope, clinical capability, and populations served.[3] Some are designed for people voluntarily seeking care who primarily need peer support and a safe place to spend the night, while others can treat people with higher acuity needs presenting with suicidal behaviors, acute agitation, and substance intoxication or withdrawal. Some are free-standing, while others are attached to or embedded in EDs or hospitals. Historically, crisis services have been financed and regulated at the state and local levels, and the absence of unifying federal oversight has contributed to the wide variability between states regarding taxonomy, licensure, and reimbursement for facility-based crisis services.

This lack of clarity poses barriers to planning and expansion efforts. Different stakeholder groups have varying expectations regarding what crisis facilities should do or whom they should serve. Existing regulations may not adequately support the creation of new types of facilities and care models. Reimbursement is often tied to provider types or whether the facility is hospital or community based. While it may be possible to shoehorn new crisis services into the existing regulatory environment, this is not ideal, because then services are created to fit artificial constraints rather than the needs of the community.

Fortunately, the momentum driving the current crisis expansion creates the opportunity to plot a course through the regulatory morass. Policymakers are working on new service definitions, standards, and payment models. At the same time, the field is rapidly evolving as communities forge ahead in creating new crisis facilities and crisis providers test new innovations.

This article is intended to support this ongoing work by providing a pragmatic framework for thinking about facility-based crisis program design that centers around the needs of people in crisis and other key stakeholders. In particular, the authors address the unique challenges of designing specialized crisis facilities that serve the full range of crises using a "no wrong door" model, including those with high acuity needs who might otherwise end up boarding in emergency departments or jail.

SERVING PEOPLE WITH HIGH ACUITY NEEDS

People with high acuity symptoms and behaviors warrant special attention when designing crisis systems. This population includes individuals who, because of a mental health and/or substance use condition, may be agitated, acutely suicidal, violent, psychotic, manic, intoxicated, and/or experiencing withdrawal. They may be involuntarily held due to posing a danger to themselves or others. This population can be the most challenging to serve, but also is the greatest in need of specialized crisis care. When the crisis continuum lacks facilities that can accommodate these high acuity needs, jails and EDs are often the only remaining options.[4] While the ED is preferred to jail, most are ill-equipped to treat people with behavioral health conditions. In a recent nationwide survey of US hospitals, only 46% of EDs reported having access to psychiatric consultation, and 59% reported that patients needing psychiatric admission must be transferred out.[5] As a result, psychiatric patients can "board" for hours or days in a setting that lacks both the expertise and environment to care for them, resulting in a poor experience for both patients and staff as well as added strain and cost on already overcrowded EDs.[6] Of particular concern, psychiatric patients are more likely to be restrained in the ED, especially those who are Black,[7] and more likely to be arrested after assaulting staff in the ED.[8]

While there is no comprehensive database of crisis facilities in the United States, the authors are concerned when they observe communities developing crisis continuums that exclude high-acuity populations. This can be due to staff anxieties about interacting with this population, concerns about whether recovery-oriented programs can employ interventions that would allow them to treat agitated or involuntary people, or involuntary processes that a community believes cannot be changed. However, if a community aspires to provide care in the least restrictive setting to all people in crisis, and reduce ED boarding and jail utilization, then policymakers must design crisis services for these high-acuity populations rather than around them.

DESIGN THINKING

The authors approach to design thinking draws from 2 existing frameworks: continuous quality improvement and architectural programming.

Continuous quality improvement (CQI) centers process and outcomes around the needs of the customer.[9] First and foremost, crisis services exist to serve people experiencing behavioral health emergencies, and thus service design must begin by clearly defining the patient population and its needs. While the patient is the primary customer, crisis systems have multiple secondary customers and stakeholders whose needs must be considered as well, such as first-responders, emergency departments, and payers.

Architectural programming emphasizes the importance of clearly articulating the problem to be solved before designing solutions.[10] Programmers work with stakeholders to define the problem by analyzing customer wants, needs, facts, and constraints. Once the problem has been clearly stated, there may be multiple design approaches that solve the problem. While this method was developed for physical spaces, the same principles provide a useful framework for the design of clinical services and processes as well.

Thus, rather than provide a set of static guidelines and definitions, this article will instead discuss how to approach facility and clinical program design around the needs of the person in crisis, key stakeholders, and the community crisis system at large. By first understanding the problems the facility needs to address, answers to questions such as staffing, process flow, and facility capabilities follow. There may be different tactics to solving a given problem, and while the authors reference existing models, their hope is that this approach supports the development of new innovations as the field of crisis care continues to evolve.

MATCHING SERVICES TO ACUITY

A fundamental value of a crisis system is to connect people with the care they need in the least restrictive setting that can safely meet their needs. This concept of least restrictive care is enshrined in the US Supreme Court's *Olmstead* decision and is consistent with what people experiencing behavioral health emergencies say they want from crisis services.[11] (In recent years, the more consumer-friendly "least intrusive" has begun to supplant this term.) Ideally, a crisis system should have a broad continuum that ranges from high-intensity programs that can serve people with the most acute needs to lower intensity programs providing peer support in home-like settings.[3]

The more comprehensive the continuum, the better the system can match services to needs throughout the course of a person's crisis. When the needed level of care does not exist, disposition defaults to the higher level of care. For example, a person who presents to the ED for suicidal ideation could potentially be stabilized in a 23-hour observation unit, but if none exists they will be admitted to an inpatient unit. In a different system that does include a 23-hour observation unit, a person may improve in this less-restrictive setting such that they can safely continue their stabilization in a lower intensity crisis residential unit. If no such crisis residential setting exists, and the patient is not yet stable enough for discharge, they will be admitted to an inpatient unit. Thus, a more robust continuum of care not only serves individuals in the least-restrictive setting but also can decrease the demand for more costly and scarce levels of care.

In a crisis continuum, it is critical that system stakeholders have a clear understanding of the capabilities of each component facility and the population it can safely serve. Lack of a shared understanding can lead to unsafe conditions (eg, when a person with high acuity symptoms and behaviors is sent to a facility that is unable to safely address their needs), delays in treatment (eg, disputes over whether a facility should accept a referral), and ineffective system planning (eg, creating a system unable to serve certain levels of acuity).

The Level of Care Utilization System (LOCUS)[12] and the American Society of Addiction Medicine (ASAM) Criteria[13] are 2 existing frameworks for assessing a person's level of acuity and describing the intensity of services needed to meet that level of acuity for mental health and substance use needs, respectively. Each uses a multidimensional approach to determining acuity, and then describes service intensity in terms of care environment, staffing, clinical services, and support services. For crisis services, these frameworks may provide a helpful starting point to describe differences in the level of medical and nursing involvement needed in various care settings.

The LOCUS assesses need across 6 dimensions: risk of harm; functional status; medical, addiction, and psychiatric comorbidity; recovery environment (both level of stress and support); treatment and recovery history; and engagement and recovery status. Facility-based services typically fall under LOCUS level 5 or 6, both of which have a subcategory for short-term crisis-focused services. Level 6 A (high-intensity, acute medically managed residential programs) includes inpatient-level care with 24/7 nursing and medical availability. Level 5 A (intensive, short-term medically monitored residential services) includes short-term residential care and includes a range of medical and nursing involvement. The final assessment synthesizes these dimensions to guide decision-making. For example, someone who expresses suicidal ideation may be able to be managed in a crisis residential setting (LOCUS level 5A) if they are highly engaged, hopeful that treatment will be helpful, and nonviolent. Conversely, an individual with suicidal ideation may require a higher acuity setting like 23-hour observation (LOCUS level 6A) if they are poorly engaged, impulsive, and highly agitated.

The ASAM Criteria include the following 6 dimensions: intoxication, withdrawal, and addiction medications; biomedical conditions; psychiatric and cognitive conditions; substance use-related risks; recovery environment interactions; and person-centered consideration. In particular, the risk of withdrawal (dimension 1) is important to consider when determining the level of medical and nursing capability required in a crisis facility. ASAM level 4 (medically managed inpatient) requires withdrawal management services that typically are available only in general hospitals and intensive care units, while ASAM level 3.7 (medically managed residential) includes community-based residential settings with 24/7 nursing and medical availability. ASAM level 3.5 (clinically managed high-intensity residential) is sometimes colloquially referred to as "social detox" or "sobering." These programs have a medical director, and they may have nursing on site for a few hours during the day with a physician on-call, but their oversight is focused on ensuring there are processes for identifying individuals in need of a higher level of medical and nursing care and arranging transfer to a more appropriate setting. ASAM level 3.1 (low-intensity clinically managed residential) has clinical services with no medical director, while a recovery residence (ASAM level RR) has no clinical services and provides a substance-free environment in a home-like setting.

In this article, the authors build off these frameworks and incorporate other considerations unique to the crisis setting. **Fig. 1** depicts common types of crisis programs along a continuum of LOCUS and ASAM level.

CORE GOALS AND CAPABILITIES OF ACUTE CRISIS CARE

Twenty-five years ago in this same journal, Michael Allen wrote an article in the Emergency Psychiatry issue which outlined the need for specialized care for people presenting to the ED in psychiatric crisis.[14] In it, he describes most psychiatric emergency services as operating with a "service under siege" culture due to overwhelming demand, and thus employing a *triage model* focused on rapid evaluation, containment, and referral. Allen advocates for a shift toward a more organized *treatment model* which includes a comprehensive assessment and a broader range of treatment options with the goals listed as follows:.

- *Improved access to care;*
- *Improved assessment*, to include a biopsychosocial formulation, differential diagnosis, and initial treatment plan, and reassessment(s) as needed during the course of the visit;

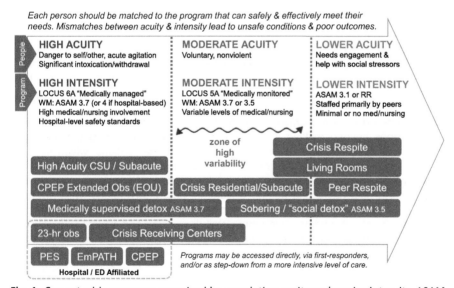

Fig. 1. Current crisis programs organized by population acuity and service intensity. ASAM, American Society of Addiction Medicine Criteria; CPEP, comprehensive psychiatric emergency program; CSU, crisis stabilization unit; ED, emergency department; EmPATH, emergency psychiatric assessment treatment and healing; EOU, extended observation unit; LOCUS, level of care utilization system; PES, psychiatric emergency services; RR, recovery residence; WM, withdrawal management.

- *Prompt initiation of definitive treatment*, which leads to reductions in symptoms, morbidity related to seclusion and restraint, and length of stay;
- *Diversion to the community*, to provide care in the least-restrictive setting, including referral pathways for step-down to community alternatives to hospitalization after the patient has been assessed and partially treated;
- *Continuity of care*, to include linkage with community provider agencies, timely appointments, and transfer of information;
- *Specialized care*, including the capability to treat youth, older adults, people with co-occurring substance use disorders (SUD), diverse language needs, and cultural backgrounds;
- *Cost effectiveness.*

These tenets still hold true, and many have been incorporated into the acute crisis programs depicted in **Fig. 1**. Some additional core elements, learned over the past 25 years, include the following:

- *Engagement and peer support:* Peer support has developed over the past several decades into a distinct and vital part of the interdisciplinary care team model. In acute crisis settings, peers are particularly skilled at engagement, de-escalation, and linkage to community resources.[15]
- *Person-centered approach:* A welcoming and inclusive program serves all populations via processes that are culturally competent and trauma informed, using recovery-oriented approaches such as shared decision-making.
- *Integrated SUD and mental health assessment and treatment*: Many if not most individuals presenting for acute crisis care have co-occurring mental health and SUD needs, and at the time of initial evaluation it is often impossible to definitively determine which symptoms and behaviors are due to substances, mental illness, or both. Thus, staff must be proficient in assessing and treating both simultaneously, and continuously adjust the diagnosis and treatment plan based on ongoing reassessments over time.
- *Specialized therapeutic milieu:* Specialized care requires specialized spaces. A safe and therapeutic milieu encompasses the physical features of the space (eg, layout, safety features such as anti-ligature fixtures, design features that create a calming environment) as well as the staff operating within the space and their roles.
- *Enhanced discharge planning:* A more holistic approach to discharge planning that goes beyond making a follow-up appointment maximizes the likelihood the person will be successful. Discharge-related interventions, which may be delivered by the crisis program or via partnerships with other community agencies, include assistance with social drivers of health, post-crisis transitional care and help navigating complex systems, brief interventions while awaiting long-term linkage, and follow-up contacts. This issue includes an article that discusses post-crisis aftercare in more detail.[16]
- *Collaboration with local system partners:* Good working relationships with system stakeholders (eg, law enforcement, EDs, provider organizations, advocacy groups, social services agencies) support CQI efforts to ensure the program is meeting community needs.

From "Medical Clearance" to Medical Stability

The American Association for Emergency Psychiatry, an organization composed of both psychiatrists and emergency medicine physicians, recommends a shift away from the vague and unhelpful term "medical clearance." Instead, a *medical evaluation* is performed to determine whether the patient is *medically stable* for treatment in a crisis facility (ie, the behavioral health symptoms are not likely due to a medical condition, and ongoing treatment for any co-occurring medical conditions is within the scope of the crisis facility).[17]

As a general rule, crisis facilities should be able to care for people who, if not for their behavioral health crisis, would be discharged home from the ED. Acute crisis facilities that provide medically managed withdrawal treatment should already have the medical and nursing capability to perform a basic medical evaluation and treat minor medical conditions (eg, asymptomatic hypertension, elevated blood sugar, urinary tract infections). Transfers to the ED can be further minimized with creative solutions such as telemedicine consults, part-time primary care coverage, etc. Crisis units embedded within an ED (eg, Emergency Psychiatric Assessment, Treatment, and Healing [EmPATH] or psychiatric emergency services [PES] units) may be able to care for higher acuity medical needs.

Acute crisis facilities should not require all individuals to undergo a "medical clearance" visit in the ED prior to arrival at the crisis facility, as this undermines the goal of avoiding unnecessary ED visits.[3] Rather, crisis facilities, EDs, first responders, and other stakeholders should work together to develop clear admission criteria and protocols for identifying medical conditions that require evaluation and treatment at an ED. Some ED-embedded crisis units may require flow through the main ED. Similarly, the goal should be timely transfer to the specialized crisis unit while minimizing unnecessary testing. Both embedded and free-standing units should engage with their stakeholders in a collaborative quality improvement process to address disagreements, delays, and suboptimal outcomes.

RECEIVING FUNCTION: RAPID DROP-OFF WITH A "No WRONG DOOR" POLICY

Compared to medical emergencies, behavioral health emergencies are unique in that the default first responder has historically been law enforcement rather than emergency medical services (EMS). While clinical response models like mobile crisis are steadily growing, police are likely to remain involved for the foreseeable future, especially in situations deemed unsafe for civilian teams and where statute requires law enforcement to transport people on an involuntary hold. This makes law enforcement a particularly important customer because they are also the first point of entry into the criminal legal system and have a choice between taking the person to jail versus a health care facility. This decision point is a critical lever for diverting people to treatment instead of jail,[18] and addresses a structural inequity that contributes to the over-incarceration of people with behavioral health conditions, especially people of color.[4] The concept of a *receiving center* was developed to incentivize law enforcement to choose treatment by making the process quick and easy.[19]

The requirements for receiving centers were first outlined as a core element of the Crisis Intervention Team (CIT) model and are listed in **Box 1**.[20] CIT, developed in Memphis, Tennessee, in the 1980s after the shooting of a Black man with schizophrenia, is a partnership between law enforcement and community stakeholders centered around improving the response to people in crisis.[21] Officers receive training on recognizing and de-escalating behavioral health emergencies, and receiving facilities provide an easy mechanism to connect the person to treatment instead of arresting them or waiting hours in the ED.

Although initially developed for law enforcement, the concept of a receiving center is applicable to all individuals in need of crisis care. Crisis facilities should provide easy

> **Box 1**
> **Crisis Intervention Team model emergency mental health receiving facility requirements[20]**
>
> "A designated Emergency Mental Health Receiving Facility is a critical aspect of the Crisis Intervention Team (CIT) model. It provides a source of emergency entry for consumers into the mental health system. To ensure CIT's success, the Emergency Mental Health Receiving Facility must provide CIT Officers with minimal turnaround time and be comparable to the criminal justice system. The facility should accept all referrals regardless of diagnosis or financial status. Additionally, the facility will need access to a wide range of emergency health care services and disposition options, as well as, alcohol and drug emergency services. Finally, the Emergency Mental Health Receiving Facility is part of the operational component of the CIT Model that provides feedback and engages in problem solving with the other community partners, such as Law Enforcement and Advocacy Communities."
>
> 1. Single Source of Entry (or well-coordinated multiple sources)
>
> 2. On Demand Access: Twenty-Four Hours/Seven Days A Week Availability
>
> 3. No Clinical Barriers to Care
>
> 4. Minimal Law Enforcement Turnaround Time
>
> 5. Access to Wide Range of Disposition Options
>
> 6. Community Interface (Feedback and Problem-Solving Capacity)

entry into the behavioral health system and be able to quickly accept anyone presenting for care, whether they arrive on their own or with family or via first responders such as police, EMS, or a mobile crisis team. For those who present in the ED, there should be a smooth process for transferring appropriate patients to specialized crisis facilities, which can reduce boarding in the transferring EDs and provide patients with a higher level of care.[22]

Of the requirements listed in **Box 1**, criteria 3 (no clinical barriers to entry) and 4 (minimal turnaround time) can be particularly challenging to operationalize. Some considerations are discussed later.

Dedicated First Responder Entrance with Rapid Drop-off Process

Receiving centers must be quicker and easier for law enforcement to use compared to arresting and booking a patient into jail. A dedicated entrance allows officers to quickly access the crisis facility without delays and inconvenience (eg, due to removing weapons) and also decreases stigma for the person in crisis by preventing others from seeing them arrive with law enforcement. Other first responders (EMS, mobile crisis teams) need to rapidly return to the field as well, and EDs are similarly designed with a separate entrance and process for EMS arrivals. First-responder drop-off times should be a key performance measure with targets under 15 minutes.[23,24]

No Wrong Door/no Refusal Policy

Police officers are not clinicians and cannot be expected to make complex triage decisions regarding which crisis facility to take someone. When officers are turned away, they are discouraged from attempting diversion in the future. Therefore, the crisis center must receive individuals 24/7 with a "no wrong door" policy. If an individual arrives who may need services at another program or facility (e.g., medical evaluation, housing services, etc.), the person (or first responder) is not turned away. Rather the crisis facility staff evaluates the person, stabilizes, and arranges for a referral or transfer if needed. While it is currently unclear if or which crisis facilities may be governed by the Emergency Medical Treatment and Labor Act law, this recommended practice of accept, evaluate, stabilize, and transfer is consistent with the spirit of the law.

No Exclusions for Behavioral Health Acuity or Civil Commitment Legal Status

People presenting for care may be agitated, a danger to themselves or others, intoxicated, experiencing withdrawal, and/or on an involuntary hold. These individuals are most in need of specialized care versus being sent to an ED, and thus the facility, clinical program, and staff training are designed to meet their needs (see **Box 1**).

FIRST 24 HOURS: ACUTE BEHAVIORAL HEALTH EMERGENCY CARE

The 24-hour mark is an arbitrary constraint but so ingrained into health care systems that it cannot be ignored. For licensure and payment purposes, services under 24 hours (eg, clinics, EDs, 23-hour observation) are typically considered outpatient, while services beyond 24 hours are something else (eg, inpatient, subacute, residential). This article will similarly discuss crisis services in terms of under or over 24 hours.

Under 24-hour programs provide acute behavioral health emergency care. These specialized units can be free-standing, or a distinct unit attached to or under a hospital or ED license, as depicted in **Fig. 1**. From a clinical standpoint, these facilities provide the highest level of emergency behavioral health care—it is a more intensive level of care than an inpatient psychiatric bed in the same way that the ED is a more intensive level of care than an inpatient medical bed because patients arrive at the inpatient bed having already received some level of assessment and treatment in the ED prior to admission. Length of stay is under 24 hours due to payment and licensing constraints and because emergency services must have continuous throughput to ensure on-demand access for the continuous arrival of new patients. The result is a highly acute and rapidly changing patient population with staffing and operational needs more like that of an ED than an inpatient unit. Programs providing this level of care are often called PES units, 23-hour emergency observation units, and Emergency Psychiatric Assessment, Treatment, and Healing units.

Population Served

Individuals typically meet inpatient (LOCUS 6A) medical necessity criteria (eg, danger to self or others, unable to care for self). Some may be too agitated or violent to be accepted by an inpatient unit until after they have undergone a period of treatment and stabilization. They may be acutely intoxicated or in need of medically managed withdrawal treatment (ASAM 3.7 in a community-based setting or ASAM 4 in a general hospital setting). In most communities, these individuals would typically be boarding in the ED awaiting transfer to an inpatient psychiatric bed. As described in the "receiving" section previously, many arrive directly from the field via first responders with little or no prior stabilization.

The level of care is driven by the person's clinical needs, not legal status, and thus these units should serve people on both a voluntary or involuntary basis. The legal status may change throughout the course of treatment, and it should be a quality goal to convert people on involuntary holds to a voluntary status within 24 hours, as has been observed in crisis stabilization facilities in Arizona.[25]

Clinical Model

The programmatic goals are to engage the person, assess their needs, begin treatment as soon as possible, and then, after a period of stabilization, connect them with the next level of care in the least restrictive setting that can safely meet their needs. For units embedded inside an ED, it must be emphasized that they should not simply be "holding" areas for psychiatric patients awaiting an inpatient bed; they should provide active treatment. Based on the initial assessment, an interdisciplinary team works to resolve the crisis via a variety of potential treatment interventions that may include medications, group and individual peer support, family engagement, motivational interviewing, care coordination, and help with psychosocial stressors and social drivers of health. After a period of observation and treatment, the person is re-assessed to determine disposition. With ongoing intensive treatment in a specialized milieu, many can be successfully stabilized and discharged to the community or stepped down to a less intensive crisis residential program without the need for inpatient admission.[22,25–27]

Clinical Staffing and Support Services

Like an ED, medical (psychiatric) and nursing coverage must be available 24/7. Ideally, psychiatric coverage by a psychiatrist or other appropriately supervised non-physician practitioner (NPP; eg, nurse practitioner or physician assistant) is on-site 24/7. Some coverage via telemedicine may be necessary in rural or under-resourced areas. Psychiatric evaluation must be performed as soon as possible so that treatment can begin quickly (within minutes if needed). The psychiatrist or NPP may see the person multiple times within a 24-hour period, versus once a day on a typical inpatient unit. The medical staff should be able to address both mental health and SUD needs as well as manage minor medical illnesses and chronic conditions. Community-based facilities should have the capability to perform simple laboratory tests waived under the Clinical Laboratory Improvement Amendments (CLIA) program.

Nurses are needed on site 24/7 to monitor and respond to patient needs and administer scheduled and pro re nata medication for psychiatric symptoms, withdrawal management, chronic medical conditions, and minor medical needs. They may need to administer medications immediately (within minutes) for treatment of acute agitation and should have access to an automated medication dispensing system that provides secure medication storage on patient care units and electronic tracking of controlled substances.

Other critical members of the interdisciplinary care team include

- Clinical staff (licensed and/or master's level clinicians, bachelor's level qualified mental health technicians) who perform assessments, obtain collateral information from families and natural supports, perform clinical interventions such as motivational interviewing and safety planning, and coordinate care;
- Behavioral health specialists who manage the milieu, ensure safety, and assist patients with activities of daily living; and
- Peers who use their lived experience to engage with individuals via individual and group interventions, address social drivers of health, and help with system navigation.

Security Personnel are not Included as Part of the Clinical Care Team

On clinical units, the management of acute agitation is a clinical activity that should be performed by highly trained clinical staff, not lesser trained security staff. Requests for a uniformed security presence, often driven by staff anxiety, should be limited to non-clinical areas such as the lobby and other public spaces, if at all. Crisis programs can also adopt a more holistic approach to safety. For example, a crisis center eliminated the use of security while significantly reducing assaults to staff by implementing process changes focused on reducing wait times, starting treatment earlier, and reorganizing the deployment of existing staff across the physical space.[28]

Seclusion/Restraint Capability

Seclusion and restraint are safety interventions to prevent imminent harm that should only be used as a last resort after other less restrictive treatment interventions have failed.[29] Having this capability enables facilities to accept people with high acuity symptoms and behaviors who would otherwise be taken to jail or the ED. In contrast to the ED, where psychiatric patients are more likely to be restrained,[6] crisis facilities have the clinical staff and physical environment to provide de-escalation and treatment instead. Staff should receive rigorous training in de-escalation, and management should implement robust quality oversight that tracks data on use and identifies opportunities for improvement. With such an approach, restraint rates can be comparable to national averages for inpatient psychiatric units.[30]

Specialized Therapeutic Milieu

The concept of a therapeutic milieu has been a mainstay of inpatient psychiatric treatment since the 1700s when French psychiatrist Phillipe Pinel observed that asylum patients were less violent when they were free to move around.[31] Milieu therapy considers the total environment—the physical space and the interpersonal interactions that occur within it—to have therapeutic value. Core therapeutic functions include containment (keeping people safe and meeting their basic needs), support (reducing stress and anxiety), structure (scheduled activities and clear staff roles), involvement (active interaction with staff and other patients), and validation (recognizing individual needs such as needing to be alone).[32] While research on milieu therapy in under 24-hour settings is lacking, the value can be intuited by comparing the experience in the ED, where patients spend hours alone in a room or on a gurney monitored by a non-clinical sitter or security guard, versus a specialized unit with room to walk around, structured groups, peer support, and ongoing therapeutic interactions with clinical staff.

Physical plant considerations for creating a safe and therapeutic milieu in the acute under 24-hour setting include

- Space that facilitates continuous observation of a high-acuity population, so that staff can monitor each individual and quickly intervene if needed.
- Space that facilitates interpersonal interaction.
- Private spaces for individual interviews, family meetings, groups, etc.
- Private spaces for physical examinations.
- Spaces that prevent overhearing clinical conversations about other people (clinical rounds, staff phone calls with families and clinics, etc.).
- Spaces that allow people, with appropriate monitoring for safety, to be away from overstimulation.
- Therapeutic and healing environment (eg, natural light, outdoor space, noise abatement, use of color and artwork, etc.).
- Capability to serve meals and snacks, launder street clothes, bathe/shower, and store personal belongings.
- Inpatient-level standards for anti-ligature safety and furnishings.
- Secured egress to prevent elopement of people on an involuntary hold.
- Capability for seclusion/restraint.
- Ability to accommodate temporary surges in volume
- Maximize staffing efficiencies (eg, avoidance of hallways and blind corners that require multiple staff to maintain line-of-sight)

Many under 24-hour programs employ an open design to accommodate observation, interaction, and temporary surges in volume. Rather than individual rooms, people are in a common space and assigned a recliner that can fold flat for sleeping, with smaller rooms available for individual clinical conversations or quiet time away from overstimulation. Approaches differ on nursing station enclosures. Some have an open nursing station area to facilitate staff-patient interaction, but staff will need to leave the area to have confidential conversations. Other units have a plexiglass barrier that allows physicians, nurses, and clinicians to remain together and in sight of the milieu with designated staff (eg, peers and techs) always stationed outside the barrier for continuous observation and interaction with patients.

BEYOND 24 HOURS: HIGH-ACUITY CRISIS STABILIZATION

While many individuals can be stabilized within 24 hours, others remain in need of care in a secure, intensive, highly monitored environment. Some would have short lengths of stay on an inpatient unit—for example, patients who are noticeably improving but are not yet stable for discharge or need more time to metabolize substances contributing to their psychiatric presentation. For this population, admission to an inpatient facility can be avoided by continuing treatment in a high-acuity crisis stabilization unit.

These units are similar to inpatient units in terms of medical necessity, staffing, physical plant, and clinical program, but with an emphasis on peer support and linkage to community-based care. It is secure, with 24/7 nursing care on-site, and daily contact with the psychiatrist or NPP, and can serve people on both a voluntary or involuntary basis with a goal of conversion to voluntary status. The average length of stay is typically under 5 days. Programs providing this level of care are sometimes referred to as "Crisis Stabilization Units, Extended Observation Units, 72-hour beds, or Short-Term Inpatient Units."

LOWER ACUITY CRISIS PROGRAMS

Not everyone in crisis needs the intensive level of care described earlier. Those able and willing to seek and engage in treatment voluntarily can and should be served in lower intensity crisis facilities. Having these services available improves the ability of the system to provide care in the least restrictive setting, providing a better experience for the person in crisis, and more judicious use of resources. However, it is important to have clear criteria and processes for assessment and referral to ensure that people are directed to programs that can safely serve them. Specific considerations include the level of agitation or behavioral acuity that can be managed in the facility, level of psychiatric and nursing support, and capability for withdrawal management.

Living Rooms and Crisis Residential Programs

Lower intensity crisis programs serve individuals who need a supportive recovery environment and are non-violent, not at imminent risk of self-harm, and able to engage in care voluntarily (LOCUS 5A). They tend to be unlocked, less institutional, more home-like (some are in actual houses), and staffed primarily with peers and behavioral health clinicians.[33] For individuals needing withdrawal management, some may provide medically monitored detox (ASAM 3.7) while others with less medical and nursing involvement may provide clinically managed "sobering" or "social detox" (ASAM 3.5). Lengths of stay can vary from under 24 hours (living rooms) to a few days to weeks (crisis residential and detox). These programs can prevent or shorten inpatient admissions by serving as stepdown from more acute treatment services such as EDs, inpatient units, and acute crisis facilities.

Urgent Care and Walk-In Crisis Clinics

Even in an urgent situation, it is not at all uncommon for waits on the order of a month or more to see a therapist and often longer for a psychiatrist. Crisis clinics offer same-day or walk-in access for outpatient assessment, crisis counseling, medication management, care coordination, and bridge services until the person is connected to appropriate outpatient care. They are typically staffed with a psychiatrist or NPP and social services staff but may also include other team members such as peer supports or financial eligibility specialists. Length of stay is typically 2 to 4 hours. These programs may function as the front door to a higher acuity unit so that people who self-present will be able to be served in either the urgent care setting or, when a higher level of care is needed, can be admitted to a 23-hour observation unit or similar setting. Without this level of care, needs may go unmet until the situation escalates to require a higher level of care.

MEASURING QUALITY AND OUTCOMES

Quality measures show whether an organization is living up to its stated values and whether the services it provides are providing value to its customers and stakeholders. The authors have previously described an approach to developing metrics for facility-based crisis services using a tool designed to help an organization translate values and customer needs into discrete measures.[23] An updated version of these measures is shown in **Fig. 2**. This issue includes an article on quality measurement that provides a more detailed discussion on the selection and application of quality measures at both the program and system level.[34]

DISCUSSION

As with other essential community services, policymakers designing crisis systems must think about the entire population of people in need of behavioral health emergency care within a given geography—including all levels of acuity, co-occurring

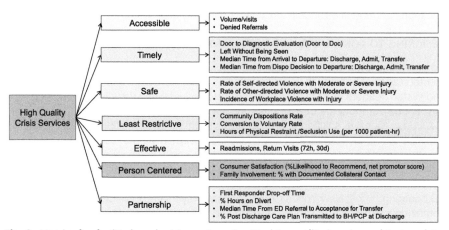

Fig. 2. Metrics for facility-based crisis services. A critical-to-quality tree is used to translate values into discrete metrics for behavioral health crisis services. (Balfour ME, Tanner K, Jurica PJ, Rhoads R, Carson CA. Crisis Reliability Indicators Supporting Emergency Services (CRISES): A Framework for Developing Performance Measures for Behavioral Health Crisis and Psychiatric Emergency Programs. Community Ment Health J. 2016;52(1):1-9. https://doi.org/10.1007/s10597-015-9954-5.)

needs (medical, SUD, etc.), and payers—and then collaborate with the relevant stakeholders to create systems and processes that ensure everyone gets the care they need in the least-restrictive setting. The National Council for Mental Wellbeing *Roadmap to the Ideal Crisis System* report includes background, guidance, and tools to support this work.[3] Later the authors discuss considerations for ensuring access to quality facility-based crisis care for high-acuity populations.

RECEIVING DIFFERENT LEVELS OF ACUITY

Receiving facilities must be able to accept all walk-ins and first-responder drop-offs without turning anyone away. Thus, it follows that receiving facilities need to contain a program or set of programs that can provide treatment to individuals of any acuity and/or a mechanism to connect them with the level of care they need. This is analogous to the trauma center model—to accept patients with any kind of injury, a Level 1 trauma center must have a set of services that can meet a variety of patient needs (trauma bay, operating room, intensive care unit, etc.) or protocols to safely transfer to a higher level of care (eg, regional burn center).

Can a receiving center function without the ability to treat people with high acuity needs? Yes, but downstream processes and outcomes will be affected, and the community will need to adjust expectations accordingly. Officers and other first responders would need to make triage decisions regarding where to bring people. Where will they take people with high acuity symptoms and behaviors? The ED? If so, then stakeholders must understand that some psychiatric patients will continue to be routed to the ED and possibly board there. Inevitably someone with high acuity needs will present for services. The facility must have clear processes for identifying when this occurs and protocols for what to do. Are they transported to a higher acuity crisis facility? How are they transported safely? Are they transported by law enforcement? That would undermine the goal of minimizing law enforcement involvement. Similarly, what happens when people with lower acuity needs present at high-acuity crisis facilities? Ideally, facilities should be designed with a mix of both higher and lower acuity services on site. If not, what are the processes to assess and refer to a lower acuity program? These are the questions communities should ask when designing their systems.

DESIGNING TO COMMUNITY AND POPULATION NEEDS

Communities have different needs, strengths, and gaps and are at different developmental stages of building their crisis systems. Thus, there is no one-size fits all solution and system leaders must take all of these into account when deciding how to structure the various components of their crisis system.

A comprehensive solution is a crisis facility that includes multiple levels of care, as depicted in **Fig. 3**. Individuals of any acuity are accepted via the receiving function, and flow through different levels of care based on their acuity and improvement over time in a single, seamless episode of care. Studies of free-standing facilities employing this model in Arizona and California show decreases in inpatient utilization, ED visits, and ED boarding.[22,25,26] New York's Comprehensive Psychiatric Emergency Program model combines a similar set of services (Triage and Referral Visit, 23-Hour Observation, and Extended Observation) into a single program that is typically attached to a hospital ED.[35]

Rural communities may lack the volume and workforce needed to sustain a free-standing crisis facility staffed to accept all individuals 24/7. Rural EDs, however, do accept all patients 24/7. A specialized unit (eg, 23-hour observation, EmPATH) attached to an ED can take advantage of the economies of scale to sustain a 24/7 nursing presence with psychiatric coverage through a mix of on-site and telemedicine

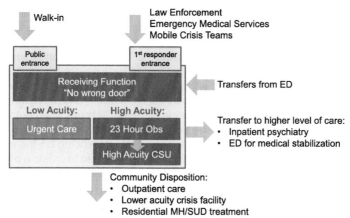

Fig. 3. Comprehensive crisis facility with multiple levels of care.

(**Fig. 4**). Many can be stabilized in the specialized unit within 24 hours.[27] For those who need ongoing care, an existing behavioral health provider that already offers outpatient and residential care might similarly maximize economies of scale by co-locating a crisis residential unit and urgent care clinic within their campus.

ED-affiliated units are an important component of the crisis continuum regardless of community size. There will always be patients with psychiatric needs in hospital EDs, either because they have co-occurring medical issues that required them to be taken there or because they chose to self-present there. Embedded or attached specialized units ensure these patients receive specialized care while also positively impacting ED throughput and revenue.[36]

CARE TRANSITIONS AND CONTINUITY OF CARE

Not only do individuals present for treatment with different levels of acuity, their acuity changes over time. Individuals may also present with multiple needs (eg, co-occurring mental health and SUD). As needs and acuity change, it is important to facilitate continuity of care through the crisis episode and smooth transitions through different levels of service intensity in the crisis continuum. The *Roadmap* report discusses these concepts in terms of vertical and horizontal flow.[3]

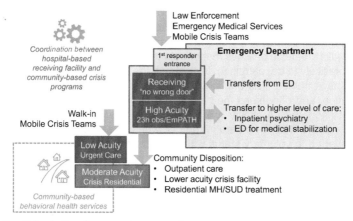

Fig. 4. Potential solution for a rural community.

Vertical flow refers to the movement through different levels of care as acuity changes over time. For example, treatment begun on a 23-hour emergency observation unit can be continued in an on-site crisis stabilization unit (CSU), a single seamless episode of care. This mitigates the inefficiencies of transfer to an off-site facility such as interruptions and delays in care, the need to duplicate psychiatric evaluations and treatment plans, opportunities for medical errors, and transportation costs. In addition, an on-site unit facilitates efficient flow through the facility and prevents individuals from becoming "stuck" on the observation unit beyond 23 hours when outside hospitals are at capacity or declining transfers due to acuity.

Care transitions to the outpatient system can differ depending on the community strengths and gaps. For example, the crisis facility might need to create a bridge clinic in a community that lacks timely access to follow-up outpatient care. Or it might partner with a community agency that already does a good job of providing post-crisis wraparound and create a process for that agency to meet with individuals before discharge for a warm handoff.

In addition, there is a need for seamless horizontal flow between various types of services for people with co-occurring mental health and SUD needs. For example, some crisis systems create distinctions between crisis beds vs. detox beds with rigid criteria regarding how each are accessed and reimbursed. Many individuals need assistance with both, and facilities should be capable of providing assessment and treatment for both. Artificial barriers should be minimized in favor of a more fluid system that meets the needs of all individuals with any combination of mental health and SUD needs.

LEAST RESTRICTIVE CARE FROM A SYSTEMS PERSPECTIVE

A core value of crisis systems is that care should be provided in the least-restrictive manner possible. As a corollary, the concept of "no force first" considers seclusion and restraints as coercive interventions to be used only as a last resort when other less restrictive methods have failed. This value must be considered from both the individual program level and the system level. At the program level, organizations should strive to minimize the use of seclusion and restraints via training, process, and quality oversight. Many crisis programs do not use seclusion or restraints at all. While this is appropriate for programs serving a lower acuity population, from a systems perspective, it is important to note that the inability to use seclusion and restraints in effect becomes the inability to accept people with high acuity symptoms or behaviors who might require seclusion or restraints. If the crisis continuum does not include a crisis facility that can accept these people, they are directed to EDs that are crowded, overstimulating, and lacking in behavioral health services, or they are taken to jail. Thus, from a systems perspective, the decision to abandon people with high acuity needs to EDs and jails creates a process that directs them to more restrictive settings where they are more likely to be restrained. In contrast, the acute crisis facilities described in this article have trained staff and physical space designed for the management of acute agitation, and oftentimes the person can be de-escalated and avoid the need for restraint altogether. A similar argument can be made for people on involuntary holds, who receive little or no care in the ED, whereas at a crisis facility the majority can be converted to voluntary status with appropriate engagement and treatment.

THE NEED FOR A COMMON TAXONOMY

The emergency medical field learned long ago that the ability to differentiate hospitals based on their capabilities is critical for developing well-organized systems of care. For example, trauma center classification into Levels I through IV provides a foundation for regional governing bodies to coordinate patient flow, geographic access, and outcome measurement. Similarly, clear understanding of the different levels of care comprising the crisis continuum would

1. Improve safety and quality of care by ensuring that people are matched to facilities that can meet their needs.
2. Support sustainable financing by providing a framework for reimbursement to reflect the intensity of the services provided.
3. Aid in organizing regional crisis systems that serve all populations—rural and urban, high acuity and low acuity, voluntary and involuntary—across a geographic region.
4. Lay the foundation for consistent licensing, accreditation, and outcome measurement.

SUMMARY

People with high acuity symptoms and behaviors present unique challenges, but specialized crisis facilities designed to meet their needs can provide care in the least-restrictive setting while minimizing unnecessary use of EDs, hospitals, and jails. The current expansion in crisis services presents an unprecedented opportunity to improve access and quality of care for people experiencing behavioral health emergencies. As communities build their crisis systems, policymakers must ensure that all populations have access to these essential services.

CLINICS CARE POINTS

- The clinical goals of acute crisis care are to engage the person, assess their needs, begin treatment as soon as possible, and then, after a period of stabilization, connct them with the next level of care in the least restrictive setting that can safely meet their needs.

- Highly agitated and involuntary individuals can be treated in specialized crisis facilities instead of the ED with appropriate staffing, clinical proceses, and physical plant design.

- The management of acuite agitation is a clinical activity that should be performed by highly trained clinical staff rather than lesser trained security staff.

- Crisis facilities should not require all individuals to undergo a "medical clearance" visit in the ED prior to referral unless there is a specific medical issue that needs evaluation.

- Crisis facilties should be able to address both mental health and substance use needs and coordinate with community providers to ensure a smooth transition to the next level of care.

DISCLOSURE

The authors have nothing to disclose.

REFERENCES

1. Substance Abuse and Mental Health Services Administration. National guidelines for behavioral health crisis care - best practice toolkit. 2020. Available at: https://www.samhsa.gov/sites/default/files/national-guidelines-for-behavioral-health-crisis-care-02242020.pdf. [Accessed 4 May 2020].
2. National Research Institute, State Profiling System, Available at: http://www.nri-inc.org/profiles/, Accessed May 25, 2024.

3. National Council for Mental Wellbeing. Roadmap to the ideal crisis system: essential elements. Measurable Standards and Best Practices for Behavioral Health Crisis Response 2021. Available at: https://www.thenationalcouncil.org/resources/roadmap-to-the-ideal-crisis-system/.

4. Balfour ME, Hahn Stephenson A, Delany-Brumsey A, et al. Cops, clinicians, or both? collaborative approaches to responding to behavioral health emergencies. Psychiatr Serv 2021. https://doi.org/10.1176/appi.ps.202000721.

5. Ellison AG, Jansen LAW, Nguyen F, et al. Specialty psychiatric services in us emergency departments and general hospitals: results from a nationwide survey. Mayo Clin Proc 2022;97(5):862–70.

6. Nordstrom K, Berlin J, Nash S, et al. Boarding of mentally ill patients in emergency departments: american psychiatric association resource document. West-JEM 2019;20(5):690–5.

7. Schnitzer K, Merideth F, Macias-Konstantopoulos W, et al. Disparities in care: the role of race on the utilization of physical restraints in the emergency setting. In: Alter HJ, editor. Acad Emerg Med 2020;27(10):943–50.

8. Disability Rights Washington. From hospitals to handcuffs: criminalizing patients in crisis. 2020. Available at: https://disabilityrightswa.org/reports/from-hospitals-to-handcuffs/.

9. Cline CA, Minkoff K. Customer-oriented continuous quality improvement: a helpful tool for improving care. first report: managed care. 2017. Available at: https://www.hmpgloballearningnetwork.com/site/frmc/content/customer-oriented-continuous-quality-improvement-helpful-tool-improving-care. [Accessed 17 March 2024].

10. Peña WM, Parshall S, Peña W. Problem seeking: an architectural programming primer. 5th edition. Hoboken, NJ: Wiley and Sons; 2012.

11. Allen MH, Carpenter D, Sheets JL, et al. What do consumers say they want and need during a psychiatric emergency? J Psychiatr Pract 2003;9(1):39–58.

12. American Association for Community Psychiatry. Level of care utilization system for psychiatric and addiction services + child and adolescent level of care utilization system. 2020. Available at: https://www.communitypsychiatry.org/locus.

13. Waller RC, American Society of Addiction Medicine. In: *The ASAM criteria: treatment criteria for addictive, substance-related, and co-occurring conditions*. 4th edition. Center City, MN: Hazelden Publishing; 2023.

14. Allen MH. Level 1 psychiatric emergency services. The tools of the crisis sector. Psychiatr Clin North Am 1999;22(4):713–34, vii.

15. Substance Abuse and Mental Health Services Administration. Peer Support Services in Crisis Care. 2022. Available at: https://store.samhsa.gov/sites/default/files/pep22-06-04-001.pdf.

16. McClanahan A, Adams CN, Hackman AL, et al. Post-Crisis follow-up and linkage to community services. Psychiatr Clin North Am 2024. https://doi.org/10.1016/j.psc.2024.04.023.

17. Wilson MP, Nordstrom K, Anderson EL, et al. American association for emergency psychiatry task force on medical clearance of adult psychiatric patients. part II: controversies over medical assessment, and consensus recommendations. West J Emerg Med: Integrating Emergency Care with Population Health 2017; 18(4). https://doi.org/10.5811/westjem.2017.3.32259.

18. Abreu D, Parker TW, Noether CD, et al. Revising the paradigm for jail diversion for people with mental and substance use disorders: Intercept 0. Behav Sci Law 2017;35(5–6):380–95.

19. Steadman HJ, Stainbrook KA, Griffin P, et al. A specialized crisis response site as a core element of police-based diversion programs. Psychiatr Serv 2001;52(2): 219–22.

20. Dupont R, Cochran S, Pillsbury S. Crisis intervention team core elements. 2007. Available at: http://www.cit.memphis.edu/information_files/CoreElements.pdf.

21. Usher L, Watson AC, Bruno R, et al. Crisis intervention team (CIT) programs: a best practice guide for transforming community responses to mental health crises. CIT International; 2019. Available at: https://www.citinternational.org/resources/Best%20Practice%20Guide/CIT%20guide%20desktop%20printing%202019_08_16%20(1).pdf.

22. Zeller S, Calma N, Stone A. Effects of a dedicated regional psychiatric emergency service on boarding of psychiatric patients in area emergency departments. West J Emerg Med 2014;15(1):1–6.

23. Balfour ME, Tanner K, Jurica PJ, et al. Crisis reliability indicators supporting emergency services (CRISES): a framework for developing performance measures for behavioral health crisis and psychiatric emergency programs. Community Ment Health J 2016;52(1):1–9.

24. Arizona Health Care Cost Containment System. Policy 590: behavioral health crisis services and care coordination. In: AHCCCS Medical Policy Manual. 2022. Available at: https://www.azahcccs.gov/shared/Downloads/MedicalPolicyManual/500/590.pdf.

25. Tomovic M, Balfour ME, Cho T, et al. Patient flow and reutilization of crisis services within 30 days in a comprehensive crisis system. Psychiatr Serv 2024. https://doi.org/10.1176/appi.ps.20230232.

26. Little-Upah P, Carson C, Williamson R, et al. The Banner psychiatric center: a model for providing psychiatric crisis care to the community while easing behavioral health holds in emergency departments. Perm J 2013;17(1):45–9.

27. Kim AK, Vakkalanka JP, Van Heukelom P, et al. Emergency psychiatric assessment, treatment, and healing (EmPATH) unit decreases hospital admission for patients presenting with suicidal ideation in rural America. Acad Emerg Med 2022; 29(2):142–9.

28. Balfour ME, Tanner K, Jurica PJ, et al. Using lean to rapidly and sustainably transform a behavioral health crisis program: impact on throughput and safety. Jt Comm J Qual Patient Saf 2017;43(6):275–83.

29. American Psychiatric Association. Seclusion or restraint. 2022. Available at: https://www.psychiatry.org/getattachment/e9b21b26-c933-4794-a3c4-01ad427eed91/Resource-Document-Seclusion-Restraint.pdf.

30. Balfour ME. Quality improvement in emergency psychiatry: the path to better outcomes and care standards. In: Glick RL, Zeller SL, Berlin JS, editors, editors. *psychiatry: principles and practice*. 2nd edition. Philadelphia, PA: Wolters Kluwer; 2019. p. 30–8.

31. LeCuyer EA. Milieu therapy for short stay units: a transformed practice theory. Arch Psychiatr Nurs 1992;6(2):108–16.

32. Gunderson JG. Defining the therapeutic processes in psychiatric milieus. Psychiatry 1978;41(4):327–35.

33. TBD Solutions. Crisis residential best practices handbook: practical guidelines and solutions. 2018. Available at: https://tbdsolutions.com/papers-presentations-2/.

34. Hopper K, Pinheiro A, Shoyinka S, et al. Multidimensional approaches to quality measurement and performance improvement in the ideal crisis system. Psychiatr Clin North Am 2024. https://doi.org/10.1016/j.psc.2024.04.002.

35. New York State Office of Mental Health. 14 NYCRR part 590 comprehensive psychiatric emergency programs guidance. 2021. Available at: https://omh.ny.gov/omhweb/bho/docs/cpep_program_guidance.pdf.

36. Stamy C, Shane DM, Kannedy L, et al. Economic evaluation of the emergency department after implementation of an emergency psychiatric assessment, treatment, and healing unit. Acad Emerg Med 2021;28(1):82–91.

Postcrisis Follow-Up and Linkage to Community Services

Alexander McClanahan, MD, MHA[a], Curtis N. Adams, MD[b],
Ann L. Hackman, MD[b], Robert O. Cotes, MD[c],
Kenneth Minkoff, MD[d],*

KEYWORDS

- Crisis care • Postcrisis follow-up • Coordination of care • Crisis stabilization
- Critical time intervention • Care-traffic control • Assertive community treatment

KEY POINTS

- The "postcrisis" period is a time of great vulnerability where individuals in crisis frequently "fall through the cracks."
- It is therefore essential for crisis systems to focus not only on front-end response, but on developing systems and services to address postcrisis needs.
- Treatment models exist that apply flexible team-based wraparound services to engage people in the postcrisis period.
- Emerging system models demonstrate how "care traffic control" and flexible funding models can facilitate system implementation of postcrisis care.
- Continuous evaluation and adaptation of postcrisis care models are vital for meeting the evolving needs of individuals and improving overall care outcomes.

INTRODUCTION

Navigating the complex landscape of mental health care, particularly for individuals and families in crisis, can often feel like walking through an unknown territory without a map. In recent years, there has been significant expansion of focus on—and resources for—the need for universal establishment of behavioral health crisis systems.[1] The implementation of 988 in July 2022 as the national Suicide and Crisis Lifeline, and

[a] Department of Psychiatry & Behavioral Sciences, Medical University of South Carolina, 67 President Street, MSC 865, Charleston, SC 29425, USA; [b] Department of Psychiatry, University of Maryland School of Medicine, 701 W Pratt Street, 5th Floor, Baltimore, MD 21201, USA; [c] Department of Psychiatry and Sciences, Emory University School of Medicine, 10 Park Place SE, Suite 620, Atlanta, GA 30303, USA; [d] ZiaPartners, Inc, 15270 North Oracle Road, Suite 124-308, Catalina, AZ 85739, USA
* Corresponding author. 15270 North Oracle Road, Suite 124-308, Catalina, AZ 85739.
E-mail address: kminkov@aol.com

Psychiatr Clin N Am 47 (2024) 531–546
https://doi.org/10.1016/j.psc.2024.04.023
0193-953X/24/© 2024 Elsevier Inc. All rights reserved.
psych.theclinics.com

a substantial focus on the implementation of mobile crisis teams, urgent care centers, and crisis centers have created significant expansion of "front-end" crisis response across the nation, as evidenced by new expectations for certified community behavioral health clinics to expand crisis services[2] as well as opportunities for states to receive increased Medicaid funding from an enhanced federal medical assistance percentage authorized by the American Rescue Plan Act.[3] However, it is becoming increasingly well recognized that behavioral health crisis episodes are not resolved with a single "one-time" intervention,[1] and that individuals and families often remain "in crisis" for an extended period following an initial crisis event. During these vulnerable periods, they may be unable to be successfully restabilized only with a "routine" referral for a "routine" outpatient appointment. Unfortunately, in the current state of behavioral health crisis system development in most communities, this critical "postcrisis" period, when people are most vulnerable and the need for continuity of care is paramount, is often characterized by inadequate service models, disconnected providers, poor communication, and a lack of systematic oversight to ensure successful transitions to downstream services.

Nonetheless, as this article will indicate, there is notable progress in developing clinical and systemic approaches to effective postcrisis behavioral health care. There is emerging recognition of the need for flexible clinical models to ensure rapid access and wraparound supports for individuals who have experienced a crisis event. At the same time, state and county behavioral health systems, as well as public and private sector payers, have increasingly recognized the crucial importance of postcrisis continuity. Some systems have endeavored to create more robust "care traffic control" and transitional care frameworks, with states like Arizona, Georgia, Missouri, and Iowa offering innovative models. Taking cues from the air traffic control industry, the most successful models prioritize meticulous tracking and adaptability. Much like how air traffic controllers ensure the safe and efficient movement of aircraft, these models focus on continually adapting to each person's needs, ensuring they are never lost in the system. However, while strides have been made, the journey is far from over. The future of postcrisis care will hinge on embracing cutting-edge technologies and fostering a patient-centered approach, where the individual's needs and experiences remain at the forefront of all interventions and strategies.

The purpose of this article is to illustrate the importance of attending to postcrisis care, describing evidence that supports successful postcrisis care services, and describe current progress in system-level care traffic control and postcrisis service funding. This information will hopefully facilitate further development of postcrisis system monitoring and service development as a necessary feature of emerging behavioral health crisis systems.

THE HANDOFF THAT IS NOT

"I came to the emergency room because I needed help. What I got was not what I expected. Eventually, I bolted because I was afraid they were going to lock me up." This is what TF, a 23-year-old man without a prior psychiatric history, said about his first experience with the mental health system. If we were to review clinical documentation from the emergency department (ED), we would see notes indicating TF had pressured speech and decreased need for sleep in the context of recent amphetamine use, and that he left against medical advice. As is commonly the case, there was no system for tracking TF and helping him reconnect, and no such connection occurred.

Four months later, TF presented to a specialized crisis care service with secure observation capacity. "When I came back, they actually did make me stay, and they gave me meds that knocked me out," he said. The notes said he presented with symptoms of mania and psychosis, stayed for 48 hours, was prescribed olanzapine, and was discharged. His only postcrisis follow-up plan was a scheduled outpatient appointment, which he never attended. Again, he was lost to follow-up. Then, 1 month later, he presented again to a crisis facility with symptoms of mania and psychosis and was restarted on olanzapine. This time a case management referral was placed. However, due to his housing instability and lack of a working telephone number, the case management team could not connect with him after discharge, and once again he did not attend the scheduled follow-up appointment. About the encounter TF later said, "They said they were going to hook me up with a case manager, but I never heard back."

Two months later, he presented again in crisis and was admitted to a psychiatric hospital for 5 days due to persistent manic and psychotic symptoms (along with continuing substance use) that did not resolve during a period of 23-hour observation. TF said, "This time, they made me stay. I had a job interview that I had to miss." Two days after hospital discharge, he was readmitted to the hospital. There, he was restarted on medication and referred to a coordinated specialty care (CSC) team for individuals with early psychosis who engaged with him while on the unit. He left the inpatient unit after 10 days and entered a supported housing program offered by the CSC team upon discharge.

Finally, 9 months after initially presenting with mental health symptoms, he attended his first outpatient appointment, had more stable housing, and was connected to CSC services. When asked about the CSC team, TF said, "I wasn't sure if anyone could help, but maybe we're getting somewhere now." It was fortunate that no seriously adverse event (eg, suicide or arrest) occurred during that period. It was also fortunate that he kept coming back in crisis to provide opportunities to help him.

When reviewing pathways from crisis to postcrisis care, hearing perspectives like TF's are not uncommon. He did not connect to outpatient care despite an ED visit, a crisis care center visit, a case management referral, and an initial inpatient hospitalization. The barriers to connection included a combination of logistical and practical barriers (eg, lack of transportation, unstable housing), inability of various systems to appropriately coordinate or provide oversight, and failure of the system to have routine access to appropriately flexible and intensive wraparound interventions after a crisis. Fortunately, in this situation, TF had access to resources that are not available in all systems, like access to CSC and being able to enter a supportive housing program quickly. These factors likely played a role in limiting the delay in making it to an outpatient appointment to only 9 months after presentation with initial symptoms.

The perspectives of people with lived experience should be a starting point to understanding these issues. Qualitative interviews of people with serious mental illness (SMI) suggest that reasons for disengagement include a lack of trust, believing one did not need services, and a mismatch between services desired versus those offered.[4] Reflexively offering an outpatient appointment without a clear explanation or goal as to how outpatient treatment can help likely will not result in a successful connection.

Based on data from the 2021 National Survey on Drug Use and Health, 52% of adults with SMI perceived an unmet need for mental health services in the past year.[5] A literature review found that disengaged individuals were more likely unsatisfied with services, felt like they were not listened to, and could not participate in decision-making processes.[6] Clearly, the way in which people experience these systems matters, and the system design for postcrisis services should emphasize responsiveness to the customers, rather than somehow expecting people in crisis to fit into the framework that is most "routine" for providers and payers.

The evidence suggests that those most in need may be most likely to fall through the cracks. Certain groups, like people experiencing first-episode psychosis, co-occurring substance use disorders and SMI, and homelessness, may require multifaceted approaches to successfully engage.[7] Although state-of-the-art crisis care facilities can often prevent inpatient hospitalization, follow-up rates from inpatient to outpatient settings remain low. In 2021, national rates of follow-up within 7 days after an inpatient mental health hospitalization ranged from 29.1% to 38.4% for people with Medicare or Medicaid and were approximately 48% for those with private insurance.[8] Furthermore, those without a prior connection to mental health resources are less likely to connect to follow-up services after a crisis. In a study of over 18,000 individuals who received inpatient services in New York State, those with less outpatient engagement prior to admission were less likely to follow up with outpatient services.[9] This lack of connection may be even more problematic among young people. In a nationwide study of individuals aged 12 to 27 years, the 7-day follow-up rate was 42.7% and 28.6% for those who had an inpatient hospitalization and ED visit, respectively, with the study again finding that those without established providers were less likely to follow up.[10]

Falling through the cracks may have significant consequences, as individuals are often vulnerable after a crisis. Systematically understanding the barriers and challenges at each stage of the care encounter may help systems develop strategies to increase the odds of individuals successfully connecting to postcrisis services. Participation in postcrisis services should never be taken for granted or assumed. The mental health system was fortunate to have multiple opportunities to welcome and engage TF in services, yet we are not always so fortunate. It is important to underscore that 35% of individuals with SMI in the United States receive no mental health treatment over the course of a year.[5] Thus, when some of the most vulnerable individuals present for services, the window may be very narrow to engage them. Each encounter matters and there might not be a second opportunity. Many individuals who experience these gaps and delays are far less fortunate than TF and wind up experiencing significant adverse outcomes, including premature death, without ever being engaged in care.

The stakes are high, and the effort to engage people in postcrisis care should be an active process undertaken by the mental health system, not just initially but in an ongoing way. Outcomes are poorer without follow-up, and unfortunately, there are few standards or expectations for developing such a system. We argue certain system-wide interventions could have connected someone like TF to care earlier. Some of these interventions include routine care traffic control tracking for anyone who presents in crisis, an expectation for the ED or crisis staff to flag someone as needing referral tracking, routine capacity for information sharing with a responsible follow-up provider, routine availability of a crisis intervention service that does intensive outreach for high-risk individuals, and routine access to transitional residential crisis services. Throughout the rest of this article, we will further describe some of the ways that systems can transform the "handoff that is not" into a successful transition to helpful and hopeful services that promote engagement and recovery.

We will start with a description of services that work, and then illustrate systemic innovations that make it more likely that—where these services exist—people in crisis will be more likely to make a successful transition and less likely to "fall through the cracks."

EFFECTIVE POSTCRISIS SERVICES—THE SERVICES THAT WORK

Let us consider another example of a person at great risk of "falling through the cracks." MX is a 28-year-old man who has been diagnosed with schizophrenia but has little awareness of his illness. He has experienced frequent ED visits and inpatient psychiatric hospitalizations and is currently unhoused. He was referred to an assertive community treatment (ACT) team from an inpatient stay because of his high service utilization but was difficult for ACT to engage or even locate because he did not have housing. His ACT psychiatrist and the team monitored his electronic medical record in an attempt to locate him. One day the psychiatrist noted that Mr X was in a nearby ED. The psychiatrist called the ED and spoke to the social worker who was attempting to arrange aftercare for MX and explained that a member of the ACT team could come to the ED to pick up MX at the time of discharge. The psychiatrist went to the ED to introduce himself and begin to engage him. MX was discharged and agreed to accept a ride from the ED to the ACT team offices. Once there, he was provided with a snack and new socks and was introduced to the ACT team's administrative staff and then to his therapist. Slowly, he began to connect with the team.

ACT is a well-known evidence-based approach for engagement and open-ended ongoing treatment of individuals with SMI who are the most seriously affected, commonly with persistent instability and recurrent crises that continue over a period of years. Many individuals experiencing a behavioral health crisis are similarly unstable and may remain unstable for a period of weeks or months and would benefit from services similar to those provided by an ACT team. However, unlike typical ACT clients, they only need that level of intensity for 30 to 90 days, not for a period of years as do most clients eligible for ACT. Is it possible to adapt what we know works from ACT to create similarly intensive but more short-term or intermediate-term team-based interventions to routinely engage individuals in the postcrisis period for weeks or months until they can transition to more routine levels of ongoing recovery-oriented treatment and support? The answer is yes.

There is an emerging literature recognizing the value of having team-based flexible application of critical time intervention (CTI) to engage individuals in the period after psychiatric hospital discharge with studies in several populations finding improved continuity of care and fewer hospitalizations.[11-13] These services have been time-limited (typically 3–9 months) and, like ACT, focus on outreach and engagement and efforts to assist individuals reintegrate into the community, develop living skills, and build support networks.[14] Behavioral health CTI has not routinely been used as part of a behavioral health crisis continuum except following hospitalization, but lends itself well to the crisis continuum particularly when CTI services borrow from the tenets of ACT providing consumer-friendly, recovery-oriented engagement strategies that help meet the needs of each person.[15] Emerging models are using these approaches as a follow-up component after mobile crisis team visits for both adults and children. The Centers for Medicare & Medicaid Services (CMS) has adopted and certain states have begun to implement a continuing crisis wraparound model for children and families called mobile response and stabilization services, which uses similar strategies.[16]

The essence of these postcrisis service models is utilizing an "ACT mentality" in the postcrisis period. ACT began a half century ago in Madison, Wisconsin, as Training in Community Living, a program designed to help people with psychiatric diagnoses whose needs were not adequately met by traditional services to develop skills necessary for living in the community. A hallmark of the model was assertive engagement[17] and this is a component essential to postcrisis team-based models using CTI. Based on the preliminary literature cited earlier, these services could be beneficial in a plethora of settings and with a variety of populations (including children and adults of all ages). This is the case with ACT, which, within 25 years, was broadly implemented in rural and urban settings, with veterans[18] and people experiencing homelessness,[19] and eventually proliferated throughout the United States and on at least

4 other continents.[20] ACT programs are currently person-centered and recovery-oriented and include not only psychiatric treatment and case management, but also employment services, housing assistance, substance use treatment, and peer services. While postcrisis CTI may not fully include all the same components as ACT, CTI can have a similarly integrated approach, and use the period of engagement to provide linkages for any type of ongoing services needed, once the person is sufficiently trusting, stable, and engaged to proceed to take advantage of those serviced.

In addition to formal components of the "ACT model," there is also a mindset ("ACT mentality"), which focuses on connecting with the people where they are and assisting them in meeting their perceived needs, which is a critical component of postcrisis CTI. Meeting the person where they are includes an ability to address a variety of needs including food, shelter, clothing, and connections in the community. Sometimes the person's perceived needs may be quite specific, but assisting them in obtaining not just a shirt but a purple shirt, and not just a sandwich but a tuna sub, with lettuce and no tomatoes from the local deli, may be invaluable in engagement and trust building. In our current fragmented behavioral health crisis system, helping get people what they want is critical, rather than simply referring them to an "appointment" that they may not even desire or see as valuable.

With this understanding in mind, key elements of postcrisis team-based CTI models include the provision of both office-based and home-based intensive care options for those who are emerging from a crisis.[21] In the initial phase of CTI, transition to the community can be accomplished by meeting a patient in an inpatient unit or in an ED to engage or reengage with them.[22] Once that connection is made, the team facilitates the second phase of CTI and helps the person make linkages to the community. Continuity of care is achieved when the CTI team helps establish or reestablish treatment and community links. In CTI, there is a transfer to longer term mental health providers (at whatever level of intensity is needed for continuing care) in phase 3 and the team can also provide rehabilitation services[23] including substance use care,[24] peer support,[15] nursing care, and somatic care.[25]

Note that postcrisis CTI follow-up services should be a "first option" for all who might be in need—that is, available to all individuals in need and not simply those who have been failed repeatedly by the system. These services should be as routinely available as "front-end" crisis services like mobile crisis teams and behavioral health urgent care walk-in centers, and these services should be available to individuals regardless of diagnosis or insurance status. It is crucial that CTI services serve children and their families and caregivers as well as adults, including older adults. CTI services should be individualized, with some needing minimal support to reconnect and move beyond the crisis and others needing much more. Whether of short or longer duration, postcrisis CTI services should be able to employ an ACT mentality (as described earlier), addressing the needs and preferences of the person or family coming for treatment, as perceived by that person or family.

Both TF and MX could also appropriately have been engaged initially with CTI services, and then connected to CSC or ACT later when they demonstrated the continuing need for those types of services. MX has been with the ACT program for almost a year now. Thus far, although MX declines antipsychotic medications and housing options, he identifies the ACT offices as his "nest." He comes somewhat sporadically to the team (the "nest") to meet with his therapist and psychiatrist, and to receive free clothing and hygiene products. He has had episodic employment with the assistance of the ACT employment specialist and while his visits to the ED have not completely stopped, they have decreased. When he does go to the ED, they point him back to the "nest" where he knows that he is welcome. This experience not only reduces expensive utilization of crisis services; it may be the difference between life and death.

CONNECTING PEOPLE TO EFFECTIVE POSTCRISIS SERVICES

Now that we have demonstrated the importance of establishing durable connections for people in a crisis and described the types of flexible, person-centered, wrap-around interventions that may be needed for people continuing to be in "crisis" following an emergency encounter, we will offer guidance on how systems can be designed to make it an expectation (rather than an exception) that these types of transitions occur. This section explores methods for enhanced "care traffic control" tracking along the crisis continuum, drawing parallels to the meticulous vigilance of air traffic control and highlighting emerging best practices from state programs and health management organizations. We will then discuss important considerations for building more robust systems.

THE "CARE TRAFFIC CONTROL" PHILOSOPHY

Ensuring adequate care for patients after a mental health crisis is an intricate task, much like the rigorous coordination required to guide an aircraft safely through a busy airspace. Each person in crisis presents with unique needs, varying problems and degrees of severity, and different socioeconomic backgrounds. Like air traffic controllers who never lose sight of their assigned aircraft, health care entities must ensure nobody becomes "lost" in the system after a crisis. The comparison, while not perfect given the inherent humanity and autonomy of someone in the midst of what may be one of their most difficult life experiences, underlines the diligence required to ensure that people in crisis do not slip through the cracks.

Many regions continue to grapple with managing people in active crisis, let alone tracking postcrisis care. However, the "care traffic control" model is showing promise. It adopts elements of the aviation industry's rigorous tracking systems, focusing on continuous monitoring along the mental health crisis continuum and ensuring proactive interventions when barriers to care arise. In this model, individual care trajectories are tracked so that health care providers can ensure a safe handoff between different levels of care, monitor clinical progress, and never lose contact.[26]

The following sections describe examples of entities or payors that have adopted elements of the care traffic control philosophy to facilitate access to intensive post-crisis services. These examples demonstrate how elements of care traffic control are being taken to scale through systemic technological advances, as well as how some systems are building service and funding models for more intensive postcrisis services. Note, however, that even a smaller community can emphasize the importance of identifying everyone who presents in an acute crisis without the latest technology and ensuring that there is an assigned responsibility to follow that person to facilitate connection to the best next step, as well as providing options for more intensive and flexible follow-up when needed, including extending the reach of existing mobile crisis services or urgent care services.

Georgia Crisis & Access Line and the Georgia Crisis & Access Line Referral Board

Georgia's Department of Behavioral Health and Developmental Disabilities pioneered a statewide 24/7 crisis hotline, the Georgia Crisis and Access Line (GCAL), that serves as the first point of contact for those experiencing a behavioral health crisis. Available to anyone in the state, GCAL connects callers to trained professionals who can assess the situation and deploy appropriate resources as needed.[27]

GCAL is complemented by the GCAL Referral Board, a cloud-based platform (developed in partnership with Behavioral Health Link, a crisis services software company) that provides a real-time snapshot of the state's behavioral health resources. This includes a comprehensive overview of all state-funded mobile crisis teams and crisis bed utilization and availability, updated in real time. Together, these components create the capacity for deploying crisis resources quickly and efficiently where they are most needed, helping to prevent emergency rooms from becoming overburdened, as well as incorporating the capacity to track information on people experiencing a crisis to promote effective "care traffic control."

The system collects essential identifying information such as name, age, gender, primary presentation, and location. It also indicates which individuals are located within each of the state's behavioral health crisis center catchment area, which ensures that resources can be allocated effectively.[28]

Moreover, the system provides flow management during the initial crisis episode and a proactive capacity to link people to ongoing care. The data system tracks each person's referral status, highlighting who is waiting for a bed, how long they have been waiting, and the current availability of beds. It is also able to schedule real-time outpatient appointments with community partners when a lower level of care is appropriate, which is an essential feature in ensuring continuity of care after a crisis event.[29] By having the 24/7 capacity to connect people with local mental health resources, and the ability to hold those local systems accountable for maintaining that availability, the system can facilitate the transition from crisis management to longer term treatment.

Arizona's Regional Behavioral Health Authority System

Arizona's Medicaid system, known as the Arizona Health Care Cost Containment System (AHCCCS), provides crisis care for all patients, regardless of their insurance status. Arizona contracts with a managed care organization in each regional behavioral health authority (RBHA) zone and sustains these services by braiding state, federal, and grant funding.[30] These entities handle a significant portion of the crisis response, including follow-up activities via phone, nonemergency transportation for crisis resolution, and emergency transport by mobile teams to crisis stabilization centers.[31] Furthermore, all AHCCCS-RBHA contractors manage crisis phone services in their areas via a unified statewide crisis helpline. Like Georgia, Arizona has incorporated a "care traffic control" approach, mandating vendors to have real-time data sharing systems across the crisis spectrum, inclusive of integrated outpatient appointment scheduling that is available 24/7 on a virtual platform to ensure access to next day follow-up for individuals in crisis as well as assigned accountability for the person served.

This system extends to the crisis recovery period, with Arizona establishing clear, proactive guidelines. Upon discharge from an inpatient unit, patients must have a scheduled follow-up appointment no later than 7 days after leaving the unit.[32] For those who interacted with the behavioral health crisis system but were not admitted, contractors must provide follow-up in-person or via telephone within 72 hours of contact.[31] This allows an additional opportunity to assess each person's risks and access to supports. Moreover, if someone faces challenges with prescribed psychotropics or experiences a change in care need, Arizona mandates the managed care organizations to actively engage with them. This proactive engagement at the systems level provides for continuous opportunities to adjust service intensity if the person in crisis is not engaging successfully in the postcrisis period.

Iowa's Crisis Stabilization Community-Based Services

Over the last decade, Iowa has made significant investments in its mental health crisis continuum, including services relating to postcrisis care. In 2014, Iowa's 99 counties were organized into 14 mental health and disability services (MHDS) regions established to provide a core set of mental health services, including 24-h access to crisis response and crisis evaluation.[33] Leveraging funding from a mixture of county mental health property taxes, state appropriations, and Medicaid,[34] Iowa further augmented its MHDS system in 2018 with legislation expanding services to include mobile response, 23-hour crisis observation and holding, residential crisis stabilization, and community-based crisis stabilization.

Crisis stabilization community-based services (CSCBSs) have allowed people to progress toward recovery after crisis in a familiar, least restrictive setting. Referrals can be made to CSCBSs directly by mobile crisis, hospital EDs, upon discharge, or through a referral line. Services among some of Iowa's CSCBSs include daily consultation with a licensed mental health professional, resiliency skill training, and connection with additional community services.[35] At least 1 regional CSCBSs has also implemented a transitional living program for patients discharged from inpatient units and in need of redeveloping skills to rejoin the community.[36]

While Iowa's CSCBS programs frequently provide services for short periods of time (7 days), crisis staff will ensure that a warm handoff has occurred to facilitate ongoing treatment. One of the key performance indicators of Iowa's CSCBS providers includes documentation of each person's progress until they can—and do—attend a follow-up appointment.[37] This is consistent with the philosophy of "care traffic control," ensuring a care entity is partnered with each person along the recovery process.

Missouri's Emergency Room Enhancement

In recent years, Missouri witnessed an alarming rate of hospitalizations for individuals with SMI, yet community-based treatment alternatives were underutilized.[38] Often these patients were uninsured or underinsured and, if not admitted from the ED, were released without a referral for follow-up services. Adding to the complexity, interactions between people with mental health issues and law enforcement often proved problematic.

These issues led the state's Department of Mental Health to launch the Emergency Room Enhancement (ERE) Program nearly a decade ago in select regions. It has since expanded to all 114 of Missouri's counties.[39] The measure is entirely funded through Missouri's Strengthening Mental Health Initiative from the Department of Mental Health[40] and focuses on linking people with significant behavioral health needs to community support. The program relies on trained hospital staff to identify those who would benefit from wraparound services and to notify ERE outreach workers. After determining the individual's eligibility, ERE staff will make an appointment with a Community Mental Health Center. Transportation will be provided if necessary. At the visit, a caseworker will provide a personalized treatment plan. Since its inception, the program has engaged over 14,000 individuals.[41] In the first 6 months of 2021, baseline measures reported a 71% decrease in homelessness, 58% reduced unemployment, and 68% and 65% reduction in ED visits and hospitalizations, respectively.[42]

In at least some regions, the success of ERE has further translated into inpatient analogs. Behavioral Health Network, the provider of ERE services for St Louis and the surrounding regions, has an embedded role in nearly a dozen hospitals. Liaisons assess the needs of admitted patients and discharge support, including follow-up phone calls, home visits, and transportation to the first follow-up appointment.[43]

USING TECHNOLOGY AND INFORMATION SHARING TO FACILITATE POSTCRISIS CONTINUITY

In addition to the specific system case examples earlier, it is important to highlight some of the more broadly applicable technology and information-sharing advances that are helping to address postcrisis continuity of care.

Crisis Notification Systems

In the continuum of postcrisis care, a significant challenge has been communication between separate systems or providers, resulting in people becoming lost in their care. This remains particularly challenging for individuals (like TF and MX) who self-present to the ED in crisis and are then discharged. This may occur because the person's level of need is not warranting an inpatient admission, but this does not mean that the person is not still experiencing significant distress and instability. Equally concerning, frequently these situations are only known within the confines of the care institution where the person presents, leading to missed opportunities for connection to resources that would provide more efficient and effective interventions. Fortunately, recent changes in health care policy and innovative technological approaches are now available that can be used by health systems routinely to improve communication and coordination in these scenarios.

The CMS took steps to address this issue with its interoperability rule, which requires certain hospitals, psychiatric hospitals, and critical access hospitals to share admission, discharge, and transfer (ADT) notifications.[44] This rule fosters open communication between health care providers, enabling better tracking of people's health status and facilitating efficient allocation of resources.

Information technology companies have partnered with providers and payors to leverage this regulatory change, developing notification systems to capture crisis events, such as ED presentations.[45] This enables care organizations to deploy proactive services, including appointment scheduling and wellness checks, for patients who need them the most, increasing their odds of navigating the recovery process. However, there remains a need to expand the use of ADT notifications in behavioral health crisis facilities, which often are not included in this hospital-based system.

Payor Discharge Collaboration

Some health maintenance organizations have begun to actively collaborate with inpatient teams to ensure patients receive timely follow-up appointments post-discharge. They have also issued comprehensive guidelines for optimizing this process, which often emphasize the identification of potential barriers to appointment attendance, such as transportation challenges and the possibility of switching to telemedicine when needed. For instance, Magellan health's guidelines stress the importance of empowering the patient to be an active participant in their care, encouraging teams to have the patient call the outpatient office while admitted to schedule the appointment. Magellan further encourages inpatient teams to promptly share the completed discharge plan so it can continue to follow the patient's progress.[46] Most other behavioral health managed care organizations are adopting similar protocols.

Building on this approach, payors can coordinate with outpatient providers to verify patient attendance at scheduled appointments and assist with rescheduling when needed. This offers an opportunity also to reevaluate the patient's care and determine if there is a need for a more intensive intervention, such as an intensive team-based CTI follow-up.

Integration of Digital Technologies

Technology and digital tools have the potential to significantly improve mental health crisis care, particularly in managing postcrisis care and ensuring that people's care trajectories are adequately tracked so they receive the follow-up care they need. The case studies explored in the previous section relied upon the implementation of technological coordination or database systems. The increasing adoption of digital health technologies, ranging from electronic health records (EHRs) to mobile health applications, also offer promising possibilities for enhancing patient engagement, continuity of care, and health outcomes after a crisis.

Integrating these digital tools and technologies into mental health crisis care could profoundly improve postcrisis management. Not only can they enhance the efficiency and quality of care, but they can also empower people who have recently been in crisis to take an active role in their health journey. However, the implementation of the following technologies should be carried out with careful consideration of data privacy and security, as well as digital health literacy among patients and providers. Ensuring equitable access to these technologies will also be critical to avoid exacerbating health disparities.[47]

Electronic health records

EHRs are integral to the effective tracking and management of patient information. They provide a comprehensive, real-time patient history that authorized health care providers across different care settings can easily access. This capability ensures continuity of care and enables providers to make informed clinical decisions based on a patient's past and current health status. For individuals post–behavioral health crises, EHRs can facilitate effective coordination among health care professionals and entities involved in their care, thus preventing them from falling through the cracks of the health care system.

Health information exchange

A health information exchange (HIE) is a system that allows the electronic sharing of health-related information among organizations according to nationally recognized standards.[48] For postcrisis care, HIE could enable seamless communication and collaboration among various entities involved in a person's care, including behavioral health specialists, primary care providers, social workers, and even family members. This capability would ensure everyone involved in a person's care is on the same page, promoting coordinated care and improving health outcomes.

Telehealth

Telehealth has emerged as an essential tool in delivering mental health services, especially amid the constraints imposed by the coronavirus disease 2019 pandemic. Telepsychiatry provides an accessible and convenient platform for people to engage with their health care providers. For postcrisis service needs, telehealth can facilitate timely follow-ups and continuous care, even when in-person visits are challenging. Many people also prefer telehealth modalities.[49,50]

Mobile health applications

The rise of mobile health (mHealth) applications has brought health care directly into the palms of consumers. mHealth apps for mental health, such as mood trackers, mindfulness apps, and therapy chatbots, offer a range of tools that can complement current services, and already some have shown benefits in managing people's symptoms for specific disorders.[51] These applications can also remind people of their appointments, assist with medication management, or provide instant support in times of distress.

These tools can be particularly beneficial in supporting selected individuals after a crisis, helping them manage their risk, and reducing the risk of an additional crisis.[52]

SUMMARY

Throughout this article, we have examined the urgent need for robust, integrated postcrisis behavioral health care, highlighting the complexity of managing people's diverse needs and the inherent challenges in coordinating and communicating between various health entities involved in patient care. We have underscored the importance of bridging gaps in care and ensuring continuity to improve clinical outcomes and reduce the chance of people reentering a state of crisis.

However, the path to realizing a seamless postcrisis mental health care system faces obstacles, such as privacy concerns, technology literacy, funding constraints, disparities in access, and the risk of technological overreliance, among others. These challenges necessitate a balanced and cautious approach to implementing change.

While this article has offered comprehensive strategies and considerations for enhancing postcrisis mental health care, the exploration should not stop here. The complexity of mental health crises, combined with the dynamic nature of health care technology and systems, demands continuous learning and adaptation. Policymakers, health care providers, and researchers must relentlessly seek novel approaches, policy modifications, and technological advancements that promote person-centric, effective postcrisis mental health care.

Furthermore, it is crucial to promote research evaluating the effectiveness of these strategies and their impact on people's quality of life, mental health outcomes, and overall health care costs. Only through such ongoing assessment and refinement can we ensure that the mental health care system meets the unique and evolving needs of every individual who seeks help in times of crisis.

In conclusion, caring for people after a mental health crisis is a daunting but surmountable challenge. With diligent effort, continuous innovation, collaboration across sectors, and a steadfast commitment to each person's well-being, we can transform the landscape of postcrisis mental health care. The stakes are high; the well-being of countless individuals hangs in the balance. But armed with knowledge, creativity, and compassion, we can make a profound difference in the lives of those affected by mental illness.

CLINICS CARE POINTS

- Seamless transition from crisis intervention to postcrisis care is essential, emphasizing the importance of immediate engagement and continuity.
- Personalized care plans, addressing the unique needs of each patient, are critical for effective postcrisis management.
- Implementing systematic care tracking and follow-up mechanisms is vital to ensure ongoing support and prevent individuals from "slipping through the cracks."
- Multidisciplinary collaboration and communication among health care providers are key to delivering comprehensive and coordinated postcrisis care.

DISCLOSURE

Outside of this work, Dr R.O. Cotes has received research funding from Alkermes, Ireland, Karuna, Otsuka, Japan, and Roche, Switzerland. He is a consultant to the

American Psychiatric Association and Saladax Biomedical, and a speaker for Clinical Care Options. The remaining authors have nothing to disclose.

REFERENCES

1. Group for the Advancement of Psychiatry. Roadmap to the ideal crisis system: Essential elements, measurable standards and best practices for behavioral health crisis response. Available at: https://www.thenationalcouncil.org/wp-content/uploads/2022/02/042721_GAP_CrisisReport.pdf. [Accessed 21 August 2023].

2. Substance Abuse and Mental Health Services Administration. Certified community behavioral health center (CCBHC) certification criteria. Available at: https://www.samhsa.gov/sites/default/files/ccbhc-criteria-2023.pdf. [Accessed 22 August 2023].

3. CMS. CMS issues guidance on american rescue plan funding for medicaid home and community based services. 2021, May 13. Available at: https://www.cms.gov/newsroom/press-releases/cms-issues-guidance-american-rescue-plan-funding-medicaid-home-and-community-based-services. [Accessed 18 January 2024].

4. Smith TE, Easter A, Pollock M, et al. Disengagement from care: perspectives of individuals with serious mental illness and of service providers. Psychiatr Serv 2013;64(8):770–5.

5. Substance Abuse and Mental Health Services Administration. Key substance use and mental health indicators in the United States: Results from the 2021 National Survey on Drug Use and Health. Available at: https://www.samhsa.gov/data/report/2021-nsduh-annual-national-report. [Accessed 21 August 2023].

6. O'Brien A, Fahmy R, Singh SP. Disengagement from mental health services. A literature review. Soc Psychiatry Psychiatr Epidemiol 2009;44(7):558–68.

7. Dixon LB, Holoshitz Y, Nossel I. Treatment engagement of individuals experiencing mental illness: review and update. World Psychiatr 2016;15(1):13–20.

8. National Committee for Quality Assurance. Healthcare effectiveness data and information set. follow-up after hospitalization for mental illness. Available at: https://www.ncqa.org/hedis/measures/follow-up-after-hospitalization-for-mental-illness/. [Accessed 21 August 2023].

9. Smith TE, Haselden M, Corbeil T, et al. The effectiveness of discharge planning for psychiatric inpatients with varying levels of preadmission engagement in care. Psychiatr Serv 2022;73(2):149–57.

10. Hugunin J, Davis M, Larkin C, et al. Established outpatient care and follow-up after acute psychiatric service use among youths and young adults. Psychiatr Serv 2023;74(1):2–9.

11. Dixon L, Goldberg R, Iannone V, et al. Use of a critical time intervention to promote continuity of care after psychiatric inpatient hospitalization. Psychiatr Serv 2009;60(4):451–8.

12. Shaffer SL, Hutchison SL, Ayers AM, et al. Brief critical time intervention to reduce psychiatric rehospitalization. Psychiatr Serv 2015;66(11):1155–61.

13. Petit J, Graham M, Granek B, et al. Pathway home™ for high utilizers of psychiatric inpatient services: impact on inpatient days and outpatient engagement. Community Ment Health J 2022;58(3):415–9.

14. Center for the advancement of critical time intervention. CTI Model. Available at: https://www.criticaltime.org/cti-model/. [Accessed 21 August 2023].

15. Salyers M, Hicks L, McGuire A, et al. A pilot to enhance the recovery orientation of assertive community treatment through peer-provided illness management and recovery. Am J Psychiatr Rehabil 2009;12:191–204.

16. Substance Abuse and Mental Health Services Administration. National Guidelines for Child and Youth Behavioral Health Crisis Care. Available at: https://store.samhsa.gov/product/national-guidelines-child-and-youth-behavioral-health-crisis-care/pep22-01-02-001. [Accessed 22 August 2023].

17. Marx AJ, Test MA, Stein LI. Extrohospital management of severe mental illness. Feasibility and effects of social functioning. Arch Gen Psychiatr 1973;29(4):505–11.

18. Valenstein M, McCarthy JF, Ganoczy D, et al. Assertive community treatment in veterans affairs settings: impact on adherence to antipsychotic medication. Psychiatr Serv 2013/05/01 2013;64(5):445–51.

19. Dixon L. Assertive community treatment: twenty-five years of gold. Psychiatr Serv 2000;51(6):759–65.

20. Rochefort DA. Innovation and its discontents: pathways and barriers in the diffusion of assertive community treatment. Milbank Q 2019;97(4):1151–99.

21. Herman D, Conover S, Felix A, et al. Critical time intervention: an empirically supported model for preventing homelessness in high risk groups. J Prim Prev 2007;28(3–4):295–312.

22. Sullivan K, Bonovitz JS. Using predischarge appointments to improve continuity of care for high-risk patients. Hosp Community Psychiatry 1981;32(9):638–9.

23. Monroe-DeVita M, Teague GB, Moser LL. The TMACT: a new tool for measuring fidelity to assertive community treatment. J Am Psychiatr Nurses Assoc Jan-Feb 2011;17(1):17–29.

24. McHugo GJ, Drake RE, Teague GB, et al. Fidelity to assertive community treatment and client outcomes in the New Hampshire dual disorders study. Psychiatr Serv 1999;50(6):818–24.

25. Vanderlip ER, Williams NA, Fiedorowicz JG, et al. Exploring primary care activities in ACT teams. Community Ment Health J 2014;50(4):466–73.

26. National Action Alliance for Suicide Prevention: Crisis Services Task Force. Crisis now: Transforming services is within our reach. Available at: https://theactionalliance.org/sites/default/files/crisisnow.pdf. [Accessed 22 August 2023].

27. Georgia Department of Behavioral Health and Developmental Disabilities. The crisis system of Georgia. Available at: https://dbhdd.georgia.gov/be-dbhdd/crisis-system-georgia. [Accessed 23 August 2023].

28. The Georgia Collaborative ASO. BHCC, CSU electronic referral and bed management [PowerPoint slides]. Available at: https://www.georgiacollaborative.com/wp-content/uploads/sites/15/2017/08/BHCC-CSU-Referral-Status-02-17-2016.pdf. [Accessed 22 August 2023].

29. Fitzgerald J. Georgia behavioral health system overview [PowerPoint slides]. Available at: https://www.house.ga.gov/Documents/CommitteeDocuments/2019/Behavioral_Health_Reform/Behavioral_Health_Reform_Commission_12.16.19_FINAL.pdf. [Accessed 23 August 2023].

30. Arizona Health Care Cost Containment System. AHCCCS FAQs: Frequent Questions About Crisis Services. Available at: https://www.azahcccs.gov/BehavioralHealth/Downloads/FrequentQuestionsAboutCrisisServices.pdf. [Accessed 23 August 2023].

31. Arizona Health Care Cost Containment System. AHCCCS Medical Policy Manual, Chapter 500 - Care Coordination Requirements. Available at: https://www.

azahcccs.gov/shared/Downloads/MedicalPolicyManual/500/590.pdf.   [Accessed 22 August 2023].

32. Arizona Health Care Cost Containment System. AHCCCS Medical Policy Manual, Chapter 1000 - Medical Management. Available at: https://www.azahcccs.gov/shared/Downloads/MedicalPolicyManual/1000/1040.pdf. [Accessed 22 August 2023].

33. Iowa Department of Health and Human Services. Regions. Available at: https://hhs.iowa.gov/mhds-providers/providers-regions/regions. [Accessed 22 August 2023].

34. Iowa Department of Health and Human Services. Issue Review: Fiscal Services Division. Adult mental health and disability services system funding history. Available at: https://www.legis.iowa.gov/docs/publications/IR/970935.pdf. [Accessed 22 August 2023].

35. Easterseals Iowa. Crisis stabilization. Available at: https://www.easterseals.com/ia/our-programs/crisis-stabilization/crisis-stabilization.html. [Accessed 22 August 2023].

36. ZION Integrated Behavioral Health Services. Services. Available at: https://zioniowa.org/services/. [Accessed 22 August 2023].

37. The Iowa Legislature. Iowa Administrative Code, section 441-24.38 (225C), Crisis stabilization community-based services. Available at: https://www.legis.iowa.gov/docs/iac/rule/10-15-2014.441.24.38.pdf. [Accessed 22 August 2023].

38. Behavioral Health + Economics Network. Forum: Improving Missouri's Crisis System: Emergency Room Enhancement Programs. Available at: https://www.bhecon.org/announcement/forum-improving-missouris-crisis-system-emergency-room-enhancement-programs/. [Accessed 22 August 2023].

39. Missouri Department of Mental Health. Emergency room enhancement program. Available at: https://dmh.mo.gov/behavioral-health/treatment-services/specialized-programs/emergency-room-enhancement. [Accessed 22 August 2023].

40. Community Counseling Center, Regional Mental Health Services. Emergency room enhancement. Available at: https://www.cccntr.com/adult-services/emergency-room-enhancement/. [Accessed 22 August 2023].

41. Missouri Department of Mental Health. FY 2022 ERE Infographic. Available at: https://dmh.mo.gov/media/pdf/fy-2022-ere-infographic. [Accessed 22 August 2023].

42. Missouri Behavioral Health Council. FY2021 Emergency room enhancement. Available at: https://www.mobhc.org/uploads/Infographic-Brief-FY2021-Q4_FINAL.pdf. [Accessed 22 August 2023].

43. Behavioral Health Network of Greater St. Louis. Hospital Community Linkages. Available at: https://www.bhnstl.org/initiatives/hcl. [Accessed 22 August 2023].

44. Centers for Medicare & Medicaid Services. Interoperability and patient access fact sheet. Available at: https://www.cms.gov/newsroom/fact-sheets/interoperability-and-patient-access-fact-sheet. [Accessed 22 August 2023].

45. Bamboo Health. Bamboo Health announces rising risk, defining the next generation of care management with real-time care intelligence. Available at: https://bamboohealth.com/press-release/bamboo-health-announces-rising-risk-defining-the-next-generation-of-care-management-with-real-time-care-intelligence/. [Accessed 22 August 2023].

46. Magellan Healthcare. Inpatient facility: Follow-up care after hospitalization leads to successful patient outcomes. Available at: https://www.magellanprovider.com/media/285533/fuh_facilitytipsheet.pdf. [Accessed 22 August 2023].

47. Rodriguez JA, Shachar C, Bates DW. Digital inclusion as health care — supporting health care equity with digital-infrastructure initiatives. N Engl J Med 2022; 386(12):1101–3.

48. The Office of the National Coordinator for Health Information Technology. Health information exchange and behavioral health care: What is it and how is it useful?. Available at: https://www.healthit.gov/sites/default/files/playbook/pdf/behavioral-health-care-fact-sheet.pdf. [Accessed 22 August 2023].

49. Yue H, Mail V, DiSalvo M, et al. Patient preferences for patient portal-based telepsychiatry in a safety net hospital setting during COVID-19: cross-sectional study. JMIR Form Res 2022;6(1):e33697.

50. Predmore ZS, Roth E, Breslau J, et al. Assessment of patient preferences for telehealth in post–COVID-19 pandemic health care. JAMA Netw Open 2021;4(12): e2136405.

51. Firth J, Torous J, Nicholas J, et al. Can smartphone mental health interventions reduce symptoms of anxiety? A meta-analysis of randomized controlled trials. J Affect Disord 2017;218:15–22.

52. Berrouiguet S, Larsen ME, Mesmeur C, et al. Toward mhealth brief contact interventions in suicide prevention: case series from the suicide intervention assisted by messages (SIAM) randomized controlled trial. JMIR Mhealth Uhealth 2018; 6(1):e8.

Clinical Practice in Crisis Services

Lessons of the Boom
A Playbook for Crisis Centers to Prevent, Survive, and Respond to Active Assailants, Targeted Violence, and Mass Violence

John S. Rozel, MD, MSL[a],*, Layla Soliman, MD[b]

KEYWORDS

- Mass shooting • Active assailant • Emergency management • Crisis services
- Behavioral threat assessment and management • Emergency psychiatry

KEY POINTS

- Crisis services may be uniquely well positioned to prevent some cases of mass violence because of the high frequency of acute and chronic stressors in the lives of assailants and crisis programs' aptitude for address those needs.
- Crisis services are uniquely well positioned to aid in immediate response and recovery to serious acts of mass violence because of their aptitude in work with acute stress and adapt to novel circumstances.
- Behavioral Threat Assessment and Management is an evidence based and effective strategy to identify and divert people at risk for serious acts for violence and is strongly complementary to general clinical and crisis care.

INTRODUCTION

What would you do with 9 seconds on a crisis telephone call? Shortly after midnight, July 20, 2012, a crisis center received a call from a man in a parking lot outside a movie theater in Aurora, Colorado. Phone records indicate that the call connected for 9 seconds. The staff member says it was a silent call that then disconnected. The caller said the call never went through. The caller later told a court appointed forensic psychiatrist that he was wondering if somebody might convince him not to carry out an attack.[1] Instead, the caller entered a movie theater, armed with 3 guns and tear gas grenades. He opened fire, killing 12 people and injuring 7 before police captured him outside of the theater.

[a] Resolve Crisis Services of UPMC Western Behavioral Health, University of Pittsburgh, 333 North Braddock Avenue, Pittsburgh, PA 15208, USA; [b] Atrium Health – Wake Forest Baptist School of Medicine, 501 Billingsley Road, Charlotte, NC 28211, USA
* Corresponding author.
E-mail address: rozeljs@upmc.edu

Psychiatr Clin N Am 47 (2024) 547–561
https://doi.org/10.1016/j.psc.2024.04.005
0193-953X/24/© 2024 Elsevier Inc. All rights reserved.

What if the call had gone through? What if the crisis clinician who answered the call had the knowledge, skills, and experience to de-escalate the caller and redirect him before he attacked the moviegoers? We can only speculate. But we know that the ongoing expansion of crisis services will mean further exposure of crisis programs to mass violence and active assailant incidents. Entwined with this exposure are needs and opportunities for crisis and emergency mental health services to enhance their capacity to recognize and help people at risk for engaging in violence.

There is a multidisciplinary field of study known as Behavioral Threat Assessment and Management (BTAM) that integrates behavioral health, legal, criminal justice, and other disciplines to understand and prevent mass attack, active assailant events, and other acts of targeted violence. One of the concepts in BTAM, also used in counterterrorism and military settings, is to distinguish "left of boom" and "right of boom," as we imagine the timeline of a mass attack.[2,3] Planning and preparation to attack (left) leads to the attack (boom), which is followed by the after-attack events (right) such as treatment of injured, prosecution, and recovery efforts.

Historically, crisis professionals primarily work right of boom: we operate family re-unification centers, Critical Incident Stress Management (CISM) intervention for first and second responders, and ongoing community support and related care. The authors propose that crisis programs have an increasingly valuable role in collaborating with other professionals to keep incidents left of boom, by identifying people at risk of violence and redirecting them from a "pathway to violence" to a "pathway to recovery."

The authors intend this article to serve as a playbook for crisis program leaders as they consider their role in preventing, managing, and responding to potential and actual attacks. It is an outline and not a comprehensive resource. These are recommendations—generously, potential best practices—and expressly neither describe nor imply a standard of care.

CRISIS SERVICES ARE UNIQUELY WELL POSITIONED TO PREVENT VIOLENCE

There is some debate about the prevalence and causal role of mental illness in mass violence; however, the trend is that mental illness is an uncommon causal risk factor.[4–6] The substantial majority of violence, it is worth reiterating, is not caused by mental illness.[7,8] Of note, there is substantial heterogeneity between studies of targeted and mass violence perpetrators in what counts as a mass shooting and what counts as mental illness playing a role in the attack making comparison between studies challenging.[9] Finally, base rates of mental illness are quite high with conservative estimates in the United States above 50% lifetime prevalence.[10] More recent studies from other economically developed countries have found lifetime prevalence by middle age 80% or above.[11,12] While there are some data to suggest that thought disorders and prior hospitalizations may be more prevalent than the general population in some data sets, they remain absent in 3 quarters of assailants.[13,14] While treating identified mental illness in a person otherwise at risk for violence can be a critical intervention, expecting to use the presence or absence or mental illness as a determinant of risk is dangerously ineffective.

Crises, on the other hand, appear to be extremely common in people who engage in serious acts of violence. There is broad consensus about the prevalence of acute crisis, trauma, and chronic stressors in the lives of the assailants. Different data sets identify the rates of acute and chronic crises from 51% to 100%.[13–16] Acute crises are often identified as precipitating and proximal risk factors for serious acts of violence, making crisis intervention a better focus for intervention than mental illness.

Community crisis programs are visible, accessible, and with a well-deserved reputation for identifying and supporting people in crisis. Some clients routinely served may be at risk for serious acts of violence, and by helping to mitigate those risk factors we may be able to reduce violence in our communities. Additionally, we can serve as an effective part of the initial evaluation and care of people newly identified as being at elevated risk for violence. Put simply, crisis services do not need to be good at predicting violence to be good at preventing violence—and this rubric is a core mantra of BTAM, a field dedicated to preventing serious acts of violence.[17]

Finally, crisis centers have historically focused on suicide prevention. The evidence of intersecting causality, etiology, and risk between violence and suicide is long standing and, again, speaks to the potential aptitude of crisis professionals in violence prevention.[18,19] According to some studies, a majority of assailants may be suicidal and about a third may die by suicide as part of their attack; other studies indicate that people who make serious threats of violence are more likely to kill themselves than somebody else.[13,20,21]

LEFT OF BOOM: PREVENTING VIOLENCE BY HELPING PATIENTS AND PREPARING YOUR TEAM FOR SERIOUS VIOLENCE

During normal operations, unless your crisis center is responding to a current attack or the immediate aftermath, you are left of boom. Mass attacks have been increasing in frequency and active shooting incidents are becoming tragically routine but both are still low base rate events. Most people who seek crisis services and have significant risk factors for violence or suicide will engage in neither. Typical interventions that mitigate risk factors relating to acute crises will also increase patients' quality of life and have the potential to reduce the risk of violence despite the difficulty of predicting violent behavior.

There is much to be said for interventions like Stop the Bleed, tactical responses to active shooters, and Run, Hide, Fight. These interventions together only work if an attack is underway. In one incident in Dayton, Ohio, 9 people were killed and 17 were injured in less than 30 seconds.[22] Waiting for the shooting to begin to have a useful tool to mitigate risk is foolhardy. Preventive strategies are imperfect, as are interventions, but together they add to the layers of proverbial Swiss cheese protecting against risks and harms.[23]

Opportunities and Limitations of Planning

Planning for potential disasters is a critical element of emergency management. Crisis center leaders should develop written plans for responding to serious acts of violence in their community and in their facility. Planning and preparation includes both the design of a plan and tabletop or actual exercises to test and refine those plans. Even when events unfold differently than imagined during planning and response training, there is still value in preparation. Planning and response exercises facilitate mid-stream adaptation because the exercises teach teams identify and adapt to potential needs on the fly during an emergency.

Further, planning and exercises should be coordinated with community partners and stakeholders—first responders including patrol and special response law enforcement, homeland security and emergency management government groups, affiliated hospitals, and other community partners. Collaboration during preparation strengthens relationship and trust during actual events. Relationship building through planning, exercises, events, and recovery is essential to effective emergency management.[24]

Planning de novo or developing new partnerships mid-disaster is not impossible and is also not ideal. In part, this is because critical incidents do not always lend themselves to careful, reflective thinking. Similarly, the experience of working relationships improves team responsiveness during real world events. Cognitive biases and errors increase under duress—and managing an unexpected serious threat, being in the midst of an ongoing shooting or hostage situation, or working in the aftermath of a shooting can exert considerable duress.[25]

Understanding and Using Behavioral Threat Assessment and Management

BTAM is broadly considered a best practice for the prevention of targeted and intentional violence.[16,26] It blends concepts and tools from behavioral science and criminal justice and uses structures and processes from the intelligence community to better understand and work with uncertainty and risk. BTAM provides a valuable tool for identifying people at risk for serious acts of violence and mitigating their risk. BTAM also highlights valuable concepts that support better clinical care and management of "routine" violence risk outside of mass-casualty threats.

BTAM is an evidence-based, ethical practice which has been developed over decades. It is also highly congruent with fundamental clinical and crisis intervention principles including a recovery orientation, emphasis on individualized assessment and treatment planning, and fostering positive interactions with natural supports and community resources. Readers aspiring to integrate BTAM into their clinical work are referred to more in-depth study[26–28] and are encouraged to engage with their local chapter of the Association of Threat Assessment Professionals (https://www.atapworldwide.org/).

Federal agencies are increasingly seeking to educate, engage, and partner with mental health professionals in BTAM work. Federal Bureau of Investigation field offices often form working relationships with local mental health practitioners as part of the FBI's Behavioral Analysis Unit's National TATM Initiative, which focuses on building local BTAM infrastructure; a substantial number of the mental health partners are crisis and emergency mental health professionals. The Department of Homeland Security offers both educational resources through the National Threat Evaluation and Reporting Program and grant funding for local BTAM-related efforts through the DHS Center for Prevention Programs and Partnerships. The US Secret Service's National Threat Assessment Center helps disseminate their research and guidance on targeted violence and mass attacks through research reports, trainings, and case analyses.

Information Sharing

Good clinical work and good threat management require collaboration and coordination of care. Routine cases as well as elevated risk threats benefit routinely from integrating input and resources, stepping outside of traditional clinical silos. Nuanced understanding of rules governing protected health information is critical to risk mitigation.

Identifying people at risk for violence often invokes duties to warn or protect third parties, but those duties vary by state and directly impact allowable disclosures of protected health information. Developing a careful understanding of these duties in your jurisdiction is often entwined with the development of a constructive relationship with legal counsel.[29]

It should be noted that the privacy regulations of the Health Insurance Portability and Accountability Act (HIPAA) allow for information sharing with law enforcement and other parties who may be able to assist in the prevention of serious acts of violence, especially in emergency situations.[30,31] Written records—but not observations, opinions, or verbal communications—are protected under the Family Educational Rights and Privacy Act (FERPA). FERPA protected information can be released by a parent or legal guardian for minors, by the student themselves once they are 18, under certain exceptions including imminent safety concerns such as major threats, and to certain types of threat management teams.[32] Crisis care situations involving imminent risk of suicide or violence often fall within the HIPAA emergency exceptions. Clinicians should use their judgment in what may be relevant or useful and disclose only the minimum protected health information needed to mitigate the threat.

Other agencies or individuals may approach crisis clinicians to give or obtain information about a client. In addition to caveats about sharing information, it should be noted that HIPAA and other health care confidentiality rules allow us to receive information without a release from the patient—and good clinical judgment should compel us to do so. This can often occur without confirming or denying that a patient is known to the clinician. While receiving information about a patient from some sources, such as law enforcement, may create some ethical challenges, these are likely to be less severe than the implications of ignoring useful information about a potentially high-risk situation.

Planning

Good emergency management practices involve routinely considering an array of potential events, their likelihood, and the range of operational impact. Active shooter incidents within a crisis facility are low likelihood, high impact events. Community based, low casualty violence that does not directly intersect the crisis service or staff is higher likelihood, lower operational impact. Apportioning resources for response and prioritizing which scenarios to spend additional time and money to prepare for can be challenging. Accrediting organizations often require health care organizations to review these assessments—hazard vulnerability analysis—on an annual basis.

In addition to developing plans for mass attack or mass casualty incidents on premises, crisis leaders may also wish to consider other scenarios:

- Psychological support for staff impacted by direct and indirect incidents
- Staff emergency preparedness plan—such as planning for childcare and other needs if staff need to shelter in place or assist with emergency response beyond their typical shift
- Serious threats made by patients against persons in the community
- Direct threats against facility or staff by patients
- Direct threats against facility or staff because of intimate partner violence involving a staff member
- Incidents in the immediate vicinity of a facility which may require a temporary facility lockdown or pose a risk to staff coming to or leaving work
- Dealing with hoaxes and false alarms including investigation of, operational or legal response to, and psychological impact on staff and community
- Rapid deployment for major incidents in the community which may require extensive staff re-allocation and rebalancing across service needs (eg, operating a family reunification center after a public event)
- Preparation for an extended lockdown due to an on-site or nearby incident (most active shooter events last minutes but some incidents can lead to hours-long "hiding")
- Whatever critical incident that just happened in your community or which you saw on the news that has left you worried.

Clinical Assessment and Interventions for People at Risk

Clinical evaluation and care for people at risk for serious acts of violence has warranted numerous other writings and course offerings, and a comprehensive discussion is well beyond the scope of this article. Some essential concepts will be reviewed. Much of the evaluation of potential risk comes down to the concept of "collecting the dots to connect the dots." To wit, professionals need to accumulate an array of information about the person of interest (POI) regarding risk and protective factors, motives, grievances, capacity for violence, and potential barriers to action. No single risk factor has been identified as both sufficient and necessary for violence in isolation from other risk factors. Conversely, no single protective factor excludes the possibility of violence.

As such, skilled clinicians need to undertake a careful analysis, ideally in coordination with a multidisciplinary team of people with expertise in BTAM. Evaluation for risk of severe violence may be precipitated by an explicit and direct threat or identified risk in a person who presented for other needs. In the field of BTAM, indirect threats and indicators of serious violence risk are referred to as "leakage."[33] The steps for assessment and management, if you will, are as easy as ABCDE:

- Assess the patient as comprehensively as possible, including collateral sources, to form a biopsychosocial assessment. Admission to extended crisis residential care or acute inpatient often allows extended assessment, intervention, the opportunity for second opinions and consultation, and formulating meaningful plans for reducing violence risk.
- Build rapport with patient and those who care for them including family and immediate acquaintances who can aid with continued support and monitoring of the patient even after leaving direct care.
- Care for the patient by treating identified psychiatric conditions, amplifying existing strengths, disrupting dynamic risk factors, and bringing resources and supports into their lives.[34] Adding even a single protective factor—housing, access to care, social supports, and so forth—can reduce violence risk by nearly 50% in some patients.[35]
- Document our understanding of the short-term and long-term risks and needs and share that formulation within the boundaries of the law.
- Evaluate again when needed based on clinical or contextual events or setbacks. Neither threat management nor psychiatric treatment is ever a one-and-done intervention.

Special Issues for Phone and Text Services

As noted earlier, leakage is extremely common before acts of violence and is often a reason for a third party contact to a crisis center. There are many ways for people to report leakage or concerns of violence that they witness in friends, peers, or strangers including specialized reporting systems in many workplaces, K12, and higher education settings as well as national referral systems such as the FBI Tip Line. Crisis phone and text services can play an important role as well, even when they are not formally structured or marketed as a program to receive such information. Crisis hotlines may have added credibility or be less imposing than other referral services; many people may be concerned for themselves or the POI by directly contacting law enforcement or law enforcement-related referral services. As such, crisis phone and text teams may receive bystander reports of threats or leakage and may be seen as a credible receiver of such information. It is incumbent on crisis programs to have clear plans on how to evaluate, manage, and, when appropriate, hand off such information.

Additionally, in a modern era of "troll culture," phone and text services can be appealing targets for hoaxes (false reports of intent to engage in severe violence) and swatting (indicating an active shooting is happening in hopes of evoking a law enforcement response). All calls should be presumed legitimate until proven otherwise; however, leadership should be prepared to support clinical staff for the psychological injury of being duped by such calls. While not a topic easily studied or quantified across crisis centers, swatting and related hoaxes are more likely than bona fide mass attacks.[36,37]

Special Issues for Mobile Crisis Services

Mobile crisis teams, on their own or through formal or informal co-response with law enforcement, can be the first assessor of a person who has made a threat of violence. Often after a person has made a threat there is a need for an urgent assessment and determination of imminent risk need for hospitalization. The flexibility of a mobile crisis team allows the rapid initiation of such assessment in a setting where the person is more likely to meaningfully engage, versus being approached solely by law enforcement. Co-response models can also provide added safety for mental health responders and added authority to encourage persons of interest to engage. Mobile crisis teams can serve as intermediaries and help vouch for the trustworthiness of law enforcement as they work to engage families or bystanders who heard threats or leakage and have critical information. In addition, mobile crisis teams can serve as credible messengers by sharing resources and information about violence and violence prevention with patients and their supports.

Special Issues for Walk-In and Residential Services

Walk-in and residential crisis services allow a setting for extended evaluation and linkage that may be difficult to obtain otherwise, particularly if inpatient services are not available or not appropriate for the specific circumstances. When possible (eg, patient willing to be admitted or meets criteria for involuntary admission), there should be a low threshold to admit people—at least once—for detailed evaluation of violence risk.[34] There should also be a readiness to develop a clear formulation and plan for managing people who may use manipulative threats of violence for secondary gain.

Appropriate training for staff on lockdown procedures, communication during active shooter incidents on premises or in the immediate community, and run/hide/fight or similar responses is essential. Note that part of "running" in run/hide/fight includes leaving wounded patients and coworkers behind; this can create ethical and moral dilemmas (and injuries) in staff.[38] An alternative model specific for health care settings, secure/preserve/fight, has also been proposed.[39]

BOOM: CRISIS ENGAGEMENT DURING ACTIVE ASSAILANT EVENTS
General Considerations

Responses seldom go according to plan during serious critical incidents. Planning and exercises help but real-world events often unfold in unexpected ways. Leaders should be comfortable adapting midstream and should remember to have compassion for their colleagues and staff who have had to make similar difficult decisions.

Crisis services often play a direct role as the designated behavioral health provider in regional incident command and emergency management systems. Crisis leaders and senior staff may find themselves in incident command centers or negotiation vans during ongoing and evolving incidents. Training, experience, and accessibility are invaluable to be able to be effective in these roles.

Crisis program leaders may need to prepare their teams for unexpected scenarios or deployments during and after critical incidents. Awareness of legal rules applying to emergency and disaster response and discussion with legal advisors about potential issues and work-arounds (eg, emergency credentialing, good Samaritan protections) may be useful. Having a core playbook of tools, responses, and interventions to work from helps. Trainings should be repeated at a cadence that reflects the impact of staffing turnover, which has accelerated in many sectors during and after COVID. Trainings should be updated as evolving science and current events require.

Crisis programs should have plans for emergency notifications of staff and the ability to quickly disseminate different messages—ranging from situational alerts (eg, stay clear of a specific location) or calls for assistance (eg, all staff needed). Staff should develop and use family emergency plans when they are required to work extended hours and potentially have limited communications with their families.

CISM and Psychological First Aid both play an important role in supporting people in the immediate aftermaths of disasters and during ongoing incidents. CISM has tools that can be used throughout an ongoing incident. The interventions are complementary but not interchangeable. Strategic planning is a critical element of CISM response and helps to assure that the right interventions are used at the right times with the right populations in the right setting.[40]

During ongoing events and the immediate aftermath, crisis leaders should work with other responders to assure that media briefings adhere to best practices including limiting graphic disclosures, minimizing the naming of assailants or showing their likenesses unless they remain at large, and assuring that there is awareness of psychological responses to trauma, measures people can take for self and mutual support, and how to access formal resources.[41,42]

Finally, while crisis programs are generally intended to divert people away from emergency department utilization, a serious incident may require more focused diversion from highly impacted emergency departments and hospitals.

Special Issues for Phone and Text Services

It is unlikely that actual mass attacks would lead to initial calls to crisis centers by people directly involved in or witnessing the event; these are more likely to go to 911. As noted earlier, hoaxes and swatting calls are common and often quite convincing. Bona fide or hoax, these calls can be incredibly demanding on staff. Real or hoax calls and text conversations may need to be preserved indefinitely for potential investigation, criminal prosecution, or other litigation.

Special Issues for Mobile Crisis Services

The first consideration for crisis leaders during a real-time community event is likely locating and protecting their mobile crisis teams, assuring that they are safe and directed to avoid high-risk areas until or unless specifically requested by other first responders. Body button devices or smartphone-based panic button systems can be important tools for staff safety and geolocation. Prompting staff to call and check in as soon as is safe when they encounter major critical incidents should be part of core training and expectations.

While mobile crisis teams are mental health professionals and not equivalent to paramedic, police, and fire first-responders, they still may be in a situation where they are on scene for major incidents. Advanced guidance on what mobile teams may be expected to do if they happen to be on scene during or immediately after an active assailant or mass casualty incident—do they retreat to a safe location? Do they provide first aid? Do they "scoop and run" people to emergency departments if emergency medical services are not immediately available (an intervention which may help save lives after shootings)[43]? Mobile crisis teams do not need to have all the equipment for a mass casualty response, but basic first aid and Stop the Bleed supplies for themselves may be reasonable.

In some critical events, mobile crisis teams may be the first called to support families and survivors during extended events and before outcomes—more specifically, the identities of the people who survived and did not—are known. If this is expected to be a role in the future or on a recurring basis, planning, specialized training, and exercises will be useful.

Special Issues for Walk-In and Residential Services

As noted, crisis programs should have plans for active assailant events on premises or in the immediate vicinity of the facility. Staff should clearly understand when and how to initiate responses and how to notify coworkers and the chain of command. Security and facility design are discussed later in this article. Psychiatric emergency services and consult liaison teams should have plans in place to assist with rapid transfer of psychiatric patients from needed medical surgical beds in acute inpatient and emergency department settings to allow those facilities to accommodate patient surges from mass casualty incidents. Co-located programs that are adjacent to or embedded in medical emergency departments may be called on for immediate family support and initial psychological triage and care for survivors.

RIGHT OF BOOM: RECOVERING AFTER TRAGEDY
General Considerations

After mass shooting and active assailant incidents, there will be more people with psychological injuries than physical injuries. As a field, we are still learning how best to respond to such incidents, both in the immediate hours and days after the incident and through continued periods of recovery which extend to years.[44] Indeed the physical and psychological injuries of the survivors can last a lifetime.

Common modalities used in the immediate response include Psychological First Aid, which focuses on civilians and families, and CISM, which focuses on first and second responders. Both have broad operational acceptance and an array of tactics and strategies relevant for any population impacted by disasters and other critical incidents.

As soon as possible after high impact events, staff should be clearly reminded about self-care and staff support resources as well as directing media inquiries to leadership, and not to search medical records of people they are not currently treating. Staff may feel the urge to look up records about an identified assailant out of concern that they may have treated them or simply out of curiosity; they may also look up the records of an injured friend, family member, or coworker. The wake of a critical incident is a terrible time to have to fire good staff who made an impulsive error.

At some point during recovery, crisis teams may be called upon to provide support for memorial services that occur in the immediate wake of the incident as well as on anniversaries. Embedded within this is the potential need for crisis leaders to need to plan and manage memorializing staff or patients who may have been killed. Grieving a patient or caller who may have perpetrated a serious act of violence is especially complex and leaders should have realistic expectations of the convoluted path to recovery, or at least, to a new normal.

In addition to anniversaries, media coverage of the incident, criminal cases and civil litigation, and similar incidents in other areas may also serve as triggers for team members and community members.

Clear guidance on preservation of operational records and communication should be sought immediately from legal or risk management advisors. When assailants survive and are apprehended, criminal prosecution is inevitable and civil litigation is also frequent after serious violent incidents. Staff and leaders may become involved as witnesses or defendants. Robust partnership with legal advisors is always useful for emergency mental health leaders.[29]

As a dialectic to the potential need to keep information privileged, especially when facing potential litigation, there are also important review processes that may occur reviewing the incidents and the responses to the incidents. The first of these, often called a hotwash, occurs within several days of closing an incident command center and allows participants to identify lessons learned from the incident specifically related to the incident command and emergency management processes. After action reports are substantially more detailed and may look at pre-incident opportunities for preventing future incidents.

Report out what you can. The plural of anecdotes may not be data, but it can be extraordinarily helpful to inform those who walk this path after you. Idiographic data on past and potential assailants are an essential tool in understanding violence risk, even accepting the fact that many of these serious incidents and their perpetrators are outliers among outliers.

Special Issues for Phone and Text Services

Some evidence suggests that highly publicized mass attacks may have a contagion effect and additional attacks may occur more frequently in the 2 to 8 weeks immediately following an index event.[45] Without a doubt, crisis centers will see an influx anxious calls as the availability heuristic makes some people over-interpret previously tolerated behaviors or communications as imminently threatening. These factors tax an already stressed system. Over longer periods of time, phone and text services may find themselves partnering with local victim support and focused recovery programs to complement their responses.

Special Issues for Mobile Crisis Services

Mobile crisis teams may be called on for a variety of group support interventions, including both formal CISM interventions as well as onsite support for families and other survivors at memorial services and trials. The group of "other survivors" can be substantial: families and friends, classmates, teammates, teachers, first and second responders, hospital teams, journalists, religious leaders, and crisis professionals themselves to name a few. Ongoing support for mobile crisis teams involved in these responses is essential.

Special Issues for Walk-In and Residential Services

Even if a crisis center is not directly impacted, staff and patients may be personally connected to the incident. While it may make sense to allow live television news reports in the immediate aftermath of an incident to be viewed in the milieu, at some point the coverage is no longer discussing pertinent developments but merely rehashing known information and potentially traumatizing viewers. Finally, walk-in and residential programs may find themselves as a safe refuge for the witnesses, families, and survivors—especially around anniversaries—who continue to live in the shadow of the trauma.

PROTECTING ACCESS AND PROTECTING CLIENTS AND STAFF: CRISIS AND EMERGENCY MENTAL HEALTH SERVICES AS TARGETS

Crisis centers are not immune from the usual risks of every publicly accessible business or health provider. In addition, by virtue of their high conflict work with a small subset of patients, crisis centers may be at elevated risk of targeted threats and attacks. Adequate security is as much about culture and practice as it is about physical engineering and building design. Both are essential and neither will be effective in isolation.

As walk-in, residential, and administrative facilities are designed de novo or renovated, physical security concerns should be expressly addressed in the design process. While this may feel onerous in an era of tightening budgets and the already exacting design standards from health care accrediting organizations, it is incumbent upon crisis leaders to advocate that security needs are not ignored. While crisis center or psychiatric emergency service specific data are unavailable, active shooter and terror attacks on health care facilities appear to be increasing.[46–48] Added to this, measures to prevent and alert people about potential events are necessarily oversensitive, resulting in high rates of false alarms and vulnerability to hoaxes—which, themselves, can have substantial psychological impact on staff and communities.

Integrating security into facility design and workflows does increase costs, but it protects access as well as staff and patient safety. That clinical settings are intrinsically soft targets does not mean that leaders and designers are powerless in mitigating risk.[49] Effective design for security which also preserves accessibility and workflow should be seen as a necessary investment in staff and patient safety. Indeed, it will take conscious effort on behalf of the design team and input from clinicians and consumers to assure that the environment still feels as comfortable and welcoming as possible to people in crisis and their families while still including necessary measures to protect people and property.

It has been said in health care, that facility design allows the choice of only 2 of these elements: accessible, affordable, and secure. Crisis programs need to be accessible and secure. Optimally, facility security should be integrated throughout the vision and design process—and not treated as a post hoc add on to the budgets and architectural plans.

SUMMARY

From the initial request from the editors to the submission of our first draft, 6 months elapsed. In that span, the Gun Violence Archive identified 387 mass shootings killing 378 people and wounding 1656 more.[50] To say nothing of the survivors, families and communities scarred and changed. It is hard to calculate the number of crisis centers who have already responded and been impacted by serious acts of violence. Every incident underscores the importance of seeking opportunities to work left of boom and crisis programs are uniquely well suited to join other professionals through BTAM and related programs to prevent serious acts of targeted violence.

CLINICS CARE POINTS

- Crisis services may be uniquely well positioned to prevent some cases of mass violence because of the high frequency of acute and chronic stressors in the lives of assailants and crisis programs' aptitude for address those needs.

- Crisis services are uniquely well positioned to aid in immediate response and recovery to serious acts of mass violence because of their aptitude in work with acute stress and adapt to novel circumstances.
- Crisis services are potentially vulnerable to active assailants because of all the usual exposures of publicly accessible health services and businesses as well as added risk because of potential conflict and frequent encounters with people at risk for violence.
- No plan is perfect but planning and exercises prior to critical incidents, especially with community partners and first responders, can substantially improve response quality and team resilience.
- BTAM is an evidence-based and effective strategy to identify and divert people at risk for serious acts for violence and is strongly complementary to general clinical and crisis care.

DISCLOSURE

Dr. J.S. Rozel receives funding from the US Department of Homeland Security and the Pennsylvania Commission on Crime and Delinquency. The authors have no other disclosures.

REFERENCES

1. Reid W. A dark night in Aurora: inside james holmes and the Colorado mass shootings. New York: Skyhorse Publishing; 2018.
2. Winkler I, Brown TC. Start with Boom. In: You CAN Stop stupid: stopping losses from accidental and malicious actions. Hoboken, NJ: Wiley; 2021. p. 255–64. https://doi.org/10.1002/9781119623946.ch16.
3. Van Horne P, Riley JA. Left of bang: how the marine corps' combat hunter program can save your life. New York: Black Irish Entertainment; 2014.
4. Metzl JM, MacLeish KT. Mental illness, mass shootings, and the politics of American firearms. Am J Publ Health 2015;105(2):240–9.
5. Rozel JS, Mulvey EP. The Link between Mental Illness and Gun Violence: Implications for Social Policy. Annu Rev Clin Psychol 2017;13(1):445–69.
6. Lankford A, Cowan RG. Has the role of mental health problems in mass shootings been significantly underestimated? Journal of Threat Assessment and Management 2021. https://doi.org/10.1037/tam0000151.
7. Swanson JW. Mental disorder, substance abuse, and community violence: an epidemiological approach. In: Monahan J, Steadman HJ, editors. Violence and mental disorder: developments in risk assessment. Chicago: University of Chicago Press; 1996. p. 101–36.
8. Elbogen EB, Dennis PA, Johnson SC. Beyond mental illness: targeting stronger and more direct pathways to violence. Clinical Psychological Science 2016; 4(5):747–59.
9. Bridges T, Tober TL, Brazzell M. Database discrepancies in understanding the burden of mass shootings in the United States, 2013–2020. Lancet Regional Health – Americas 2023;22. https://doi.org/10.1016/j.lana.2023.100504.
10. Kessler RC, Berglund P, Demler O, et al. Lifetime prevalence and age-of-onset distributions of DSM-IV disorders in the national comorbidity survey replication. Arch Gen Psychiatry 2005;62(6):593.
11. Caspi A, Houts RM, Ambler A, et al. Longitudinal assessment of mental health disorders and comorbidities across 4 decades among participants in the dunedin birth cohort study. JAMA Netw Open 2020;3(4):e203221.

12. Kessing LV, Ziersen SC, Caspi A, et al. Lifetime incidence of treated mental health disorders and psychotropic drug prescriptions and associated socioeconomic functioning. JAMA Psychiatry 2023. https://doi.org/10.1001/jamapsychiatry.2023.2206.

13. Peterson JK, Densley J. The violence project database of mass shootings in the United States, 1966-2019. Saint Paul, MN: The Violence Project; 2019. Available at: https://www.researchgate.net/publication/337261684_The_Violence_Project_Database_of_Mass_Shootings_in_the_United_States_1966-2019.

14. Silver J, Simons A, Craun S. A study of the pre-attack behaviors of active shooters in the United States between 2000 and 2013. Federal Bureau of Investigation. Washington, DC: US Department of Justice; 2018. Available at: https://www.fbi.gov/file-repository/pre-attack-behaviors-of-active-shooters-in-us-2000-2013.pdf/view.

15. Brucato G, Hesson H, Dishy G, et al. An analysis of motivating factors in 1,725 worldwide cases of mass murder between 1900-2019. J Forensic Psychiatr Psychol 2023;0(0):1–14.

16. Alathari L, Drysdale D, Driscoll S, et al. Protecting America's schools: a U.S. Secret service analysis of targeted school violence. Washington, DC: U.S. Secret Service, Department of Homeland Security; 2019. Available at: https://www.secretservice.gov/sites/default/files/2020-04/Protecting_Americas_Schools.pdf.

17. Simons A, Meloy JR. Foundations of threat assessment and management. In: Van Hasselt VB, Bourke ML, editors. Handbook of behavioral criminology. Cham: Springer International Publishing; 2017. p. 627–44. Available at: http://drreidmeloy.com/wp-content/uploads/2017/12/2017_FoundationsOfThreat.pdf.

18. Plutchik R. Outward and inward directed aggressiveness: the interaction between violence and suicidality. Pharmacopsychiatry 1995;28(S 2):47–57.

19. Plutchik R, van Praag HM, Conte HR. Correlates of suicide and violence risk: III. A two-stage model of countervailing forces. Psychiatr Res 1989;28(2):215–25.

20. Active Shooter Incidents: 20-Year Review, 2000-2019. Federal bureau of investigation. Washington, DC: US Department of Justice; 2021. Available at: https://www.fbi.gov/file-repository/active-shooter-incidents-20-year-review-2000-2019-060121.pdf/view.

21. Sturidsson K, Warren L, Runeson B, et al. Mortality among offenders convicted of threatening violence: A population-based study. Journal of Threat Assessment and Management 2023. https://doi.org/10.1037/tam0000208.

22. Hassan A. Dayton Gunman Shot 26 People in 32 Seconds, Police Timeline Reveals. The New York Times. Available at: https://www.nytimes.com/2019/08/13/us/dayton-shooter-video-timeline.html. [Accessed 26 August 2023].

23. Wyman J, Cooper PW, Gibson K. The swiss cheese effect: organizational misbehavior and active threat. Orlando, (FL): Association of Threat Assessment Professionals Winter Conference; February 4; 2022. Available at: https://www.atapworldwide.org/resource/resmgr/ATAP_-_Agenda_-_8.5x11.pdf. [Accessed 26 August 2023].

24. Olszewski C, Siebeneck L. Emergency management collaboration: A review and new collaboration cycle. J Emerg Manag 2021;19(1):57–68.

25. Kleespies PM. Decision making in behavioral emergencies: acquiring skill in evaluating and managing high-risk patients. Washington, DC: American Psychological Association; 2014.

26. Behavioral Analysis Unit. Making prevention a reality: identifying, assessing, and managing the threat of targeted attacks, . Federal bureau of investigation. US

Department of Justice; 2016. Available at: https://www.fbi.gov/file-repository/making-prevention-a-reality.pdf. [Accessed 27 February 2017].

27. Meloy JR, Hoffman J, editors. International handbook of threat assessment. 2nd edition. New York: Oxford University Press; 2021.

28. Follman M. Trigger points: inside the mission to Stop mass shootings in America. 1t edition. New York: Dey St, an Imprint of William Morrow; 2022.

29. Rozel JS. Identifying and understanding legal aspects of emergency psychiatry unique to different jurisdictions. In: Fitz-Gerald MJ, Takeshita J, editors. Models of emergency psychiatric services that work. integrating psychiatry and primary care. Cham: Springer International Publishing; 2020. p. 165–75. https://doi.org/10.1007/978-3-030-50808-1_16.

30. U.S. Department of Health and Human Services, Office for Civil Rights. HIPAA Helps Caregiving Connections: HIPAA helps mental health professionals to prevent harm. 2017. Available at: https://www.hhs.gov/sites/default/files/hipaa-helps-prevent-harm.pdf. [Accessed 30 May 2022].

31. Federal Bureau of Investigation. Health insurance portability and accountability act (HIPAA) privacy rule: a guide for law enforcement. Available at: https://www.fbi.gov/file-repository/hipaa-guide.pdf/view. [Accessed 26 August 2023].

32. Does FERPA permit the sharing of education records with outside law enforcement officials, mental health officials, and other experts in the community who serve on a school's threat assessment team? | Protecting Student Privacy. U.S. Department of Education. Available at: https://studentprivacy.ed.gov/faq/does-ferpa-permit-sharing-education-records-outside-law-enforcement-officials-mental-health. [Accessed 29 January 2024].

33. Meloy JR, O'Toole ME. The concept of leakage in threat assessment. Behav Sci Law 2011;29(4):513–27.

34. Barnhorst A, Rozel JS. Evaluating threats of mass shootings in the psychiatric setting. Int Rev Psychiatr 2021;33(7):607–16.

35. Elbogen EB, Johnson SC, Newton VM, et al. Protective Mechanisms and Prevention of Violence and Aggression in Veterans. Psychol Serv 2014;11(2):220–8.

36. Enzweiler MJ. Swatting political discourse: a domestic terrorism threat. Notre Dame Law Rev 2015;90(5):2001–38.

37. Lorenzo SNR Ronald. Swatting. In: Romaniuk SN, Catino MS, Martin CA, editors. The Handbook of homeland security. Boca Raton, FL: CRC Press; 2023. p. 295–300.

38. Giwa AO, Urdaneta AE, Wedro B. Call of duty- what are physicians obligations during crises? J Emerg Med 2022;0(0). https://doi.org/10.1016/j.jemermed.2022.07.017.

39. Inaba K, Eastman AL, Jacobs LM, et al. Active-shooter response at a health care facility. N Engl J Med 2018;379(6):583–6.

40. Everly GS, Lating JM. Disaster mental health: strategic planning. In: Everly GS, Lating JM, editors. A clinical guide to the treatment of the human stress response. New York: Springer; 2019. p. 227–39. https://doi.org/10.1007/978-1-4939-9098-6_11.

41. Lankford A, Madfis E. Don't name them, don't show them, but report everything else: a pragmatic proposal for denying mass killers the attention they seek and deterring future offenders. Am Behav Sci 2018;62(2):260–79.

42. Clark DW, Volkmann P. Enhancing the crisis management briefing. Int J Emerg Ment Health 2005;7(2):133–40.

43. Jacoby SF, Reeping PM, Branas CC. Police-to-hospital transport for violently injured individuals: a way to save lives? Ann Am Acad Polit Soc Sci 2020; 687(1):186–201.
44. Allsopp K, Brewin CR, Barrett A, et al. Responding to mental health needs after terror attacks. BMJ 2019;366:l4828.
45. Towers S, Gomez-Lievano A, Khan M, et al. Contagion in mass killings and school shootings. PLoS One 2015;10(7):e0117259.
46. McNeilly B, Jasani G, Cavaliere G, et al. The rising threat of terrorist attacks against hospitals. Prehospital Disaster Med 2022;37(2):223–9.
47. Kelen GD, Catlett CL, Kubit JG, et al. Hospital-based shootings in the United States: 2000 to 2011. Ann Emerg Med 2012;60(6):790–8.e1.
48. Wax JR, Cartin A, Craig WY, et al. U.S. acute care hospital shootings, 2012-2016: A content analysis study. Work 2019;64(1):77–83.
49. Hesterman JL. Soft target hardening: protecting healthcare facilities, workers, and patients from attack. J Healthc Protect Manag: Publication of the International Association for Hospital Security 2021;37(2):65–75.
50. Mass shootings in 2023 | gun violence archive. gun violence archive. Available at: https://www.gunviolencearchive.org/reports/mass-shooting. [Accessed 1 September 2023].

Attending to Persons with Intellectual and/or Other Developmental Disorders in Crisis Settings

Lisa Anacker, MD[a], Matthew Edwards, MD[b],
Stacy Nonnemacher, PhD[c], Debra A. Pinals, MD[d],*

KEYWORDS

- Developmental disorders • Crisis settings • Crisis services • Crisis response system
- Effective communication

KEY POINTS

- Persons with Intellectual and/or Other Developmental Disorders (I/DD) exhibit difficulties along social, cognitive, and behavioral dimensions that begin to manifest during the developmental period.
- While acknowledging the heterogeneity of this group of people, individuals with I/DD nevertheless have unique needs within the crisis response system that can result in challenges for providers in crisis settings.
- Clinical considerations for persons with I/DD in crisis settings include recognizing the frequency of co-occurring medical and psychiatric disorders and being aware of this population's communication and behavioral presentations.
- Legal considerations for persons with I/DD in crisis settings can be related to safety, capacity, guardianship, and civil commitment.
- Determining if and when to engage a person with I/DD's supporters when providing crisis services is critical and can enhance the process of moving someone through a crisis and diverting future crises.

INTRODUCTION

The implementation of 988 as a new, easy-to-remember national number for crisis and suicide prevention has been a watershed moment in mental health and substance use

[a] Center for Forensic Psychiatry, 8303 Platt Road, Saline, MI 48176, USA; [b] Psychiatry, Stanford University School of Medicine, 401 Quarry Road, Suite 2204, MC 5723, Stanford, CA 94305, USA; [c] NASDDDS (National Association of State Directors of Developmental Disabilities Services), P.O. Box 26128, Alexandria, VA 22313, USA; [d] Department of Psychiatry, University of Michigan, Rachel Upjohn Building, 4250 Plymouth Road, Ann Arbor, MI 48109, USA
* Corresponding author. Department of Psychiatry, University of Michigan, Rachel Upjohn Building, 4250 Plymouth Road, Ann Arbor, MI 48109.
E-mail address: dpinals@med.umich.edu

Psychiatr Clin N Am 47 (2024) 563–576
https://doi.org/10.1016/j.psc.2024.04.024
psych.theclinics.com
0193-953X/24/

services. One of the galvanizing forces to rolling out services to match the new number has been Substance Abuse and Mental Health Services Administration's 2020 guidelines on crisis services best practice toolkit, which referenced a crisis response continuum as including "someone to call," "someone to respond," and a "safe place to go" (which is now often referred to as a "safe place to be" for youth or generically a "safe place for help").[1] As policymakers have begun to roll out an increasingly robust crisis continuum, specific populations are being recognized for their unique needs within the crisis response system, including persons with intellectual and/or other developmental disabilities.[2] This study presents information to help describe the population's needs from a biopsychosocial perspective and address crisis services specifically and how they may need to be tailored to meet those needs.

WHO ARE PERSONS WITH INTELLECTUAL AND/OR OTHER DEVELOPMENTAL DISORDERS?

Every person, regardless of their abilities, is unique, and thus there is no single way to describe persons with intellectual and/or other developmental disorders (I/DD) and what they might need from a crisis response perspective. Nonetheless, it is important to recognize that persons with I/DD are a heterogeneous group of people. There are many types of neurodevelopmental disorders. Though an exhaustive review of each of them is beyond the scope of this study, the common elements include that they exhibit difficulties along social, cognitive, and behavioral dimensions that begin to manifest during the developmental period, typically prior to early 20s, though often definitions for particular systems will be prior to age 18, 21, or 22 years, depending on what rules exist for different services or programs.

Diagnosis

Intellectual developmental disorder (IDD) is diagnosed in individuals with intellectual and adaptive functioning deficits that often manifest before a child enters grade school.[3] Historically, intellectual functioning was measured through intelligence quotient (IQ) tests, though *The Diagnostic and Statistical Manual of Mental Disorders, fifth edition (DSM-5)* de-emphasized IQ tests within the diagnostic criteria. The diagnosis no longer requires a full-scale IQ, yet this test will still typically be done to indicate intellectual functioning as part of the assessment. The diagnosis as a whole, however, now focuses more attention on the need to use clinical assessment and judgment when diagnosing IDD.[4] This could be, at least in part, because individuals with IDD with the same IQ score can still exhibit a spectrum of functional abilities. Relying on IQ score alone may result in limitations and failure to capture an individual's capabilities with respect to adaptive skills, needs, and behavioral manifestations.[5] Adaptive functioning, rather than an IQ score alone, is what typically determines the amount of support an individual with IDD may require.[3] Nevertheless, standardized test scores are still included in an individual's evaluation, and indeed, the *DSM-5* notes that persons with IDD typically score approximately 2 standard deviations or more below the population mean, which equates to an IQ score of approximately 70 or below.[3]

Instead of IQ scores being the essential factor defining a person's overall ability, the *DSM-5* suggests that an individual's level of impairment should be classified as mild, moderate, severe, or profound based on deficits of adaptive functioning in conceptual, social, and practical domains.[3] The conceptual domain includes assessment of an individual's academic skills, including reading, writing, and arithmetical, as well as a person's memory and ability to plan and problem solve.[3] The social domain includes evaluation of a person's interpersonal communication abilities, as well as their perception of social cues, awareness of others' emotions, and empathy.[3] The practical domain involves the estimation of an individual's daily living tasks and self-management activities, including feeding, personal care, money management, and organization.[3] Considered broadly, adaptive functioning compares an individual to others similar in age and background and estimates how well that person is able to meet societal standards of independence and responsibility.

A comprehensive diagnostic evaluation for IDD could include not only an assessment of an individual's cognitive and adaptive functioning but also a prenatal and perinatal medical history, a family pedigree, a physical examination, and possible genetic screening or neuroimaging. Of note, visual and hearing tests should be considered when evaluating a child for IDD, as hearing and vision difficulties can result in communication and social skills deficits, mimicking IDD.[6]

In a crisis setting, behaviors and clinical presentations of persons with I/DD can pose diagnostic challenges. Clinical presentations of individuals with I/DD may include communication difficulties, affective symptoms, psychosis, agitation, or externalizing behaviors,[7] to name a few common ones. Special consideration should be given to differentiate how intellectual and developmental disorders contribute to an individual's presentation versus primary psychiatric or behavioral disorders that may also contribute. Although the use of neuropsychological and cognitive testing can help determine an individual's developmental level and functioning, in crisis settings, this information may not be available. To the extent possible, clinicians attempting to sort through a complex clinical picture should have at the ready questions to ask staff or family about history and prior testing when they accompany the patient.

In crisis settings, it is likely that full diagnoses of IDD will not be done, but the clinician should be mindful that for a person not yet diagnosed with IDD, they may need referral for further workup. Given crisis services' goals of ensuring safety and providing timely and appropriate stabilizing care for patients in acute mental health or substance use distress, clinicians may face diagnostic limitations and constraints and may desire more information to aid their assessment than what is available to them.

Etiology and Prevalence

The causes of IDD are diverse. Although many cases of IDD are due to unknown etiology, the underlying reason for IDD is often distinguished by genetic or nongenetic causes. Genetic causes are varied and can be single gene mutations such as Fragile X syndrome, copy number variations, or chromosomal abnormalities such as Trisomy 21 or Down syndrome.[6] Genetic syndromes are more likely in individuals with severe or profound IDD.[8] Nongenetic causes of IDD can include environmental exposures, including in utero exposures to alcohol and other teratogens,[9] maternal infections, delivery complications, and postnatal trauma. It is important to help ensure, therefore, that pregnant women in crisis settings are referred for proper prenatal care and guidance to minimize any potentially avoidable causes of IDD in their children.

The prevalence of IDD is estimated at 1% to 3% of children in high-income countries.[3,8,10,11] In low-income and middle-income countries, there are some data to suggest that the prevalence of IDD may be higher, secondary to increased environmental exposures such as undernutrition and infections.[12] Most people diagnosed with IDD are classified as having mild intellectual disability.[13] Male individuals are more likely than female individuals to be diagnosed with IDD,[14] which may be explained, at least in part, by X-linked causes of the disability, such as Fragile X syndrome.[13]

Co-occurring Disorders

IDD is often intertwined and co-occurring with other neurodevelopmental disorders, psychiatric disorders, and medical disorders. Assessments of the rates of IDD and psychiatric comorbidities vary. However, studies have estimated that mental health problems in individuals with IDD can be 3 to 5 times higher compared to those in the general population.[13,15,16] Another review estimates that 40% of children and adolescents with IDD present with a mental health problem that is either diagnosed or at diagnosable levels, with the prevalence of psychiatric symptoms even higher across neurogenetic syndromes.[8] The rate of 40% is at least double that compared to children without IDD.[8] Co-occurring mental disorders are thought to be more predictive than the severity of IDD when considering a child or adolescent's restrictions related to participation in educational and vocational activities, as well as their social inclusion.[15] Co-occurring psychiatric disorders in persons with IDD can include depressive and anxiety disorders and schizophrenia, among others.[3,17,18]

Among children with IDD, approximately 18% are estimated to also meet criteria for autism spectrum disorder (ASD),[19] and approximately 39% are estimated to have attention deficit hyperactivity disorder (ADHD),[20] 2 other significant neurodevelopmental disorders. Although there remains a need for research examining substance use and addiction in persons with IDD, data suggest that those with IDD who use substances are at an increased risk for negative consequences, such as increased risk-taking and aggression.[21,22] Self-injurious behaviors and challenging behaviors also occur frequently in IDD populations.[8] Challenging behaviors, often defined as behaviors that pose a risk to the individual or others,[8] can be complex and a frequent reason that family members contact a health care professional. Deficient communication skills, combined with a possible underlying mental health problem, can present as aggressive or challenging behaviors in this population. Given the elevated rates of psychiatric disorders in this population, it is not surprising to consider that they will likely appear in crisis settings.

Medical conditions can also co-occur with IDD. Epilepsy affects 17% to 50% of persons with IDD, compared to 0.5% to 1% in the general population, with its prevalence rising as the severity of IDD increases.[13,23] Traumatic brain injury (TBI) is also comorbid at increased rates in individuals with IDD compared to the general population. Persons with IDD experienced a significantly higher risk of TBI over a 15 year period,[24] thought to be due to, at least in part, a greater risk of experiencing injuries and falls associated with factors such as comorbid epilepsy, limitations in recognizing hazards, and a greater propensity for self-injurious behaviors.[25–27] Falls were shown to be a leading contributor to TBIs in persons with IDD, similar to the general population.[24]

Health care professionals should be cognizant of the possibility of co-occurring psychiatric and medical conditions when diagnosing and treating an individual with IDD. Being aware of and identifying any co-occurring conditions can provide other targets for intervention that can result in a significant impact on the functioning of a person with I/DD. It is often people who have co-occurring I/DD and mental health conditions who have the most need for responsive and holistic support provided by skilled professionals, particularly in times of crisis.

Despite the known incidence of psychiatric disorders in the I/DD population, there has been a long-held misconception that a person with I/DD cannot have a co-occurring mental health condition.[28] This misconception often supports the practice of diagnostic overshadowing or the misattribution of symptoms of one illness to an already diagnosed comorbidity.[29] For example, some may see an individual with I/DD who is in crisis and communicating through externalizing behavior like property destruction and attribute the experience to the person's intellectual or developmental disability, rather than more appropriately to the anxiety that they are experiencing in an unknown or unfamiliar situation. This practice of diagnostic overshadowing stymies service systems and clinicians' abilities to provide the necessary holistic, person-centered supports and services often leading to an underdiagnosis of other comorbid conditions, as well as to obstacles in accessing necessary supports that may divert someone from more dire outcomes like jail or prison.

Unfortunately, service systems tend to spend time and energy attempting to identify a "primary diagnosis" with the intention of assigning a funding stream responsible for the care of the person. Due to a lack of knowledge and capacity, the mental health service system may attempt to redirect the person to the I/DD system, which may be ill-equipped to support mental health needs of the person with I/DD. The complex presentations of people with I/DD and MH conditions are less familiar to most practitioners and pose a challenge to fully understanding the person.[30] However, understanding the presentation is critically important and can be done using resources like *The Diagnostic Manual—Intellectual Disability: A Clinical Guide for Diagnosis of Mental Disorders in Persons with Intellectual Disability.*[31] Because of the prevalence of mental health conditions and the field's growing understanding of the presentation in people with I/DD, improvement in ensuring that people with I/DD receive adequate mental health care in the community, including necessary crisis services and support, is essential.[32] Personnel providing crisis response and treatment can be better equipped to support someone with I/DD if they acknowledge the comorbidity of I/DD and mental health conditions while also understanding how mental health conditions may present in this population. Crisis stabilization services should design supports and treatment that consider this co-occurrence focusing on necessary habilitative, behavioral, and psychiatric modalities.

Other Neurodevelopmental Disorders

Separate from IDD itself, it is important to take note of other neurodevelopmental disorders that can be present in individuals presenting in crisis settings. ADHD is a neurodevelopmental disorder delineated by impaired levels of attention, along with disorganization, and/or hyperactivity or impulsivity.[3] Clinicians in a crisis setting who may be seeing a youth with oppositional defiant disorder or conduct disorder should be aware that ADHD may overlap with these externalizing conditions.[3] ASD is a neurodevelopmental disorder characterized by persistent deficits in areas of social communication and interaction, along with types of restricted, repetitive behaviors that begin within the developmental period.[3] Similar to IDD, a diagnosis of ASD alone does not fully communicate an individual's functional abilities, and clinicians should be aware of the adaptive functioning of persons with ASD when identifying their capabilities and care needs. In a crisis setting, aggression and self-injurious behaviors may be common reasons for a person with ASD to present.[33] Providers should be mindful of sensory stimuli in crisis settings, as people with ASD may differ in their perception of, or responses to, environmental stimuli.[34] While not a focus of this study, other neurodevelopmental disorders can also include motor, communication, and specific learning disorders.

CLINICAL CONSIDERATIONS FOR PERSONS WITH INTELLECTUAL AND/OR OTHER DEVELOPMENTAL DISORDERS IN CRISIS SETTINGS

The crisis mental health system is tasked with the vital need to care for an increasingly diverse population. As noted earlier, intellectual and other developmental disorders impact an individual's functioning in a number of domains, including communication, understanding, reasoning, learning, and behavior.[35] Individuals with intellectual disability and other developmental disorders contribute to the diversity of clinical presentations in the crisis mental health system.

The same system challenges that impact the larger mental health system may also pose barriers to care for individuals with I/DD, though persons with I/DD may be more likely to have acute changes in behavior that lead to psychiatric emergencies and engagement with crisis services.[36] Challenges include difficulties in coordinating care across systems, decreased access to care, and limited resources. Resource limitations such as limited bed availability may increase boarding times and cause delays in care for individuals with mental illness and I/DD.[35,37] Additionally, when individuals receive care across multiple systems, clinicians may encounter incomplete medical histories of intellectual and developmental disorders. Individuals with comorbid psychiatric illnesses and some degree of cognitive impairment may be underserved by both systems, lacking the severity of intellectual and developmental disability to receive services for developmental disabilities while also relying on care in crisis settings that is poorly equipped to meet their needs.[38]

Clinicians should consider whether behaviors of a person with I/DD are functional, which is defined as behavior that "serves a purpose for the individual."[7] These situations may be shaped by behavioral reinforcement. For example, covering one's ears when encountering interpersonal conflict may be reinforced and continued over time because it helps an individual escape or avoid a particular situation.[7] These behaviors are adaptive behaviors that serve a particular (ie, desirable) function for the individual. While these behaviors are not necessarily pathologic, they can limit physical, social, occupational, or other functions or interfere with physical and psychosocial well-being.

In some cases, individuals without intellectual or developmental impairments (eg, deaf and other hard-of-hearing individuals) may be inappropriately referred to mental health or behavioral health services[30] when the impairment and the need for further supportive aids is really at issue. At the same time, such individuals may require a crisis intervention, and systems are gearing up for how to help all individuals who call for help or appear at a crisis stabilization center. Similarly, individuals with functional behaviors such as vocalization, repetition, and abnormal speech may be interpreted as psychotic. In other cases, individuals with cognitive and intellectual disabilities may mask deficits. This "cloak of competence" occurs when individuals with mild-to-moderate intellectual disability demonstrate functional and adaptive skills that belie underlying cognitive deficits.[38] Intellectual and cognitive symptoms may "overshadow" other behavioral observations.[38] Individuals with I/DD may exhibit deficits in communication that do not reflect the severity of potential co-occurring mental health symptoms. Prevalence rates of trauma among the I/DD population are known to be very high, and as such, creating a trauma-sensitive environment within the crisis service array is critical, as is diagnostic assessments.[39]

Thus, there are numerous potential challenges with ensuring that individuals with I/DD receive appropriate behavioral health treatments or interventions, just as there are challenges with recognizing the full spectrum of behaviors that might serve as barriers to individuals with co-occurring mental disorders and intellectual disabilities receiving the care they need.[38] Some of these functional behaviors may resemble behaviors commonly seen in psychiatric disorders or may place the individual or others in danger. Special care is needed in these situations to employ the best intervention for the individual in that context. Behavioral approaches offering support (eg, applied behavior analysis or positive behavioral supports) by trained clinical practitioners may be the best course to understand and treat the behavioral presentation of these individuals.

Although the purview of mental and behavioral health broadly encompasses psychiatric, behavioral, and cognitive disorders, some behavioral health clinicians receive comparatively little training in diagnosing intellectual and developmental disorders and in working to support their needs in treatment contexts. This may make these complex presentations less familiar and more challenging to understand.[30] Such complex presentations contribute to inappropriate referrals for psychiatric treatment among individuals with I/DD in crisis and other mental health settings.[40] This is significant because such individuals may be treated with medication or other interventions that are not actually indicated. These include medications such as sedatives and antipsychotics as well as environmental interventions such as seclusion and restraints. Seclusion, isolation, and restraint may contribute to distress, trauma, and mistrust of the mental health system, particularly for individuals with I/DD.

LEGAL CONSIDERATIONS FOR PERSONS WITH INTELLECTUAL AND/OR OTHER DEVELOPMENTAL DISORDERS IN CRISIS SETTINGS

Most mental health clinicians assign diagnoses based on the *DSM*, currently in its fifth revised edition. The (Diagnostic and Statistical Manual of Mental Disorders, Fifth Edition, Text Revision [*DSM-5-TR*]) includes psychiatric and behavioral disorders ranging from affective and psychotic disorders to substance use and neurocognitive disorders.[3] Although a diagnosis based on the *DSM-5-TR* does not carry statutory legal authority, most courts consider whether an individual meets clinical criteria for a diagnosis in the *DSM-5-TR* when considering legal standards that involve questions about issues such as psychiatric disability, criminal responsibility, competency to stand trial, decision-making capacity, and civil commitment. A *DSM-5-TR* diagnosis of a major psychiatric illness or intellectual and developmental disability does not alone lead to civil commitment or the determination that an individual lacks capacity but may support a court's determination that criteria are met or not met in cases when an individual's deficits, impairments, or symptoms affect specific competencies, capacities, and behaviors. As noted in later discussion, diagnoses with the *DSM-5-TR* may be limited for individuals with I/DD in that many of their symptoms of mental illness can look different or be described differently from those of people without I/DD.

In crisis settings, presentations related to safety, capacity, guardianship, and circumstances leading to consideration of civil commitment may arise. Individuals are presumed to conduct their lives and make decisions on their behalf unless there are behaviors, observations, or other factors that suggest they may lack these capacities. Individuals with I/DD may be assessed to determine whether their cognitive impairments and any co-occurring mental health symptoms interfere with their ability to make safe, reasonable, and consistent decisions, whether any co-occurring conditions are present that interfere with safe functioning or need for treatment, and whether there are any particular legal issues that may arise related to these factors.

Some individuals with I/DD may have a familial, state-appointed, or designated guardian who may serve as their decision-maker. When the person appears in a crisis setting, it is important for the clinical care team to know whether there is a guardian involved. These guardians may enter into legal and administrative decisions that affect the care and well-being of individuals with I/DD. Civil commitment raises issues for a number of populations (eg, children, criminal defendants, sex offenders, intellectual disabilities, and mental illness). Various state and federal case laws, statutes, and other procedures help shape care provisions for these individuals. In crisis contexts, states generally have laws that allow for the involuntary holding of people who meet specific criteria, such as being at risk of harm to themselves or others due to mental illness.[41] When persons with I/DD have a co-occurring mental illness, these laws may also pertain to them. Guardians may also be permitted also authorize an individual to remain in a crisis setting, depending on the state's laws.

The Americans with Disabilities Act (ADA) of 1990 broadly prohibited the discrimination of individuals with disabilities in the United States.[42] Its reach spanned labor and employment, public accommodations, education, and transportation. Federal law continues to recognize the right of individuals to live without discrimination on the basis of their disability. The Supreme Court of the United States (SCOTUS) reexamined these principles in a landmark case (*Olmstead v LC*) in 1999.[43] In its decision, SCOTUS ruled that unjustified detention of individuals with disabilities violated the ADA. It resulted in individuals residing in community settings over institutional settings when reasonable accommodations were available. The provisions today for Home and Community-Based Services (HCBS) require that persons with I/DD receiving care are living in the least restrictive and most integrated settings possible if they are receiving Medicaid funding to support them.[44] As such, when warm handoffs are occurring to community services, it is important to keep in mind these HCBS tenets.

During the 1990s, Kentucky law allowed individuals with cognitive impairment to be civilly committed when there was "clear and convincing evidence" to support civil commitment.[45] By contrast, the law required evidence "beyond a reasonable doubt" for individuals with a mental illness or disorder. Concerned citizens petitioned the court, arguing that such a double standard violated the Constitution's equal protection clause. In 1993, SCOTUS upheld the law,[45] meaning that some states may have separate civil commitment laws for persons with I/DD. Clinicians practicing in crisis settings should, therefore, be cognizant of the legal regulation or practice that can implicate persons with I/DD with and without a co-occurring mental illness.

STRATEGIES TO SUPPORT PERSONS WITH INTELLECTUAL AND/OR OTHER DEVELOPMENTAL DISORDERS IN MOBILE CRISIS SERVICES, CRISIS STABILIZATION, AND INPATIENT SERVICES

Crisis response may occur in a person's home environment when mobile crisis is dispatched, or it may occur in a crisis stabilization center or even an inpatient psychiatric unit. Existing crisis response and stabilization programs and models should consider a few nuances when developing processes and treatments for persons with I/DD. Finding ways to better understand people who may struggle with communication, engaging supporters, and understanding the impact of co-occurring mental health conditions is incredibly important to support someone with I/DD in crisis more effectively.

Effective Communication

Communication is central to assessment and treatment, especially in persons with I/DD. People with I/DD who use or need a communication tool or other supports or strategies have a lot in common, yet many have different disability, cultural, and life experiences accounting for the diversity of people who may require crisis support and services.[46] Further, times of crisis may interfere with one's ability to communicate effectively, exacerbating existing social and communication access needs someone may have,[47] or complicating communication for people who may be bilingual. This reinforces the need to utilize existing bilingual crisis supports for people with I/DD. Some strategies to incorporate into existing crisis response and stabilization services when engaging with someone with I/DD are listed in **Box 1**.

Communication is critical at every stage of crisis support. Acknowledging and creating processes that provide people with the tools, support, and strategies to effectively communicate and get their needs met should occur at every point of the crisis continuum.

Engaging Family and Caregivers

Some people with I/DD rely on family, friends, paid supporters (often referred to as direct support professionals), or others to assist in their daily lives. Any of these individuals may accompany individuals when they present in a crisis setting. Determining if and when to engage these supporters when providing crisis services is critical and can enhance the processes and treatment in moving someone through a crisis situation and diverting future crisis situations. During mobile response and stabilization, assessment is key in identifying strengths and triggers, ultimately informing the development of a crisis safety plan that focuses on positive future outcomes.[49] During this assessment process, supporters can be helpful in providing information or assisting the person in a way that they can share information about themselves that would inform the plan.

For community-based crisis stabilization services where the focus is keeping people in their community and providing behavioral health treatment like counseling and skills training, engaging the person's supporters as part of the multidisciplinary team is critical in planning for transition to their home.[50] Since some people with I/DD are being supported while living and working in their communities, people providing support can be helpful in reminding, reinforcing, and coaching the person to generalize skills and strategies to their daily lives in hopes of managing future potential crises. One would expect that these supporters can also generalize these approaches and become part of the continuum in preventing crisis for that person with I/DD. A person's community support system can be a great asset to divert a person with I/DD from crisis services and transition them back to their community living, supporting the national goal of creating crisis services that are for "anyone, anywhere, and anytime."[51] It is important to note that engaging with supporters should always be at the discretion of the individual and taking the time to ensure that the person is comfortable with including a particular supporter is essential.

Box 1
Facilitating effective communication with persons with intellectual and/or other developmental disorders in crisis and stabilization services

- Build rapport and trust through providing an introduction and finding common interests to anchor the discussion

- Minimize use of open-ended questions; consider "either/or" questions

- Assess for understanding to ensure the person with I/DD is not acquiescing or repeating what they have heard or what they think others want them to say

- Use short, simple sentences—avoid jargon

- Rephrase words and questions and provide examples as necessary

- Provide ample response time[48]

Medication and Behavioral Approach to Crisis Care for Persons with Intellectual and/or Other Developmental Disorders

The complex and co-occurring presentations of individuals with I/DD may contribute to inappropriate treatment with medication that is not actually indicated in an acute setting. Prescribing antipsychotic, mood stabilizing, or sedative medication to reduce a presenting behavior such as aggression may lead to unintended, long-term consequences for the health of the individual with I/DD. Collaboration and communication with primary treating providers may help crisis staff identify whether a medication is indeed appropriate and, if so, which medication has helped the individual in acute settings in the past. More research into evidence-based interventions relating to medication and individuals with I/DD in crisis is warranted.

It is essential to understand that a person with I/DD may be engaging in a behavior (eg, aggression) as a symptom of their mental health condition or to serve a function or purpose. This understanding is critical to crisis services' determination of the best approach for their support and treatment.[52] For example, after careful assessment and observation, it may be noted that a person with I/DD who has a co-occurring schizophrenia diagnosis becomes aggressive toward their roommate without provocation or trigger. In this case, one may consider whether the aggression is a symptom of schizophrenia, perhaps in response to a delusion, if the aggression does not appear to serve a behavioral purpose such as an attempt to get their roommate's attention. While a good behavioral approach focuses on crisis prevention, in crisis service settings, determining if the behavior is serving a function can be done through a functional behavior assessment (FBA). An FBA is a systematic process of identifying problem behaviors and the events that predict the occurrence of the behaviors that maintain the behaviors across time.[53] Immediate crisis situations like outreach to call centers do not always afford this type of systematic assessment, but this can be a referral for ongoing stabilization after the immediate crisis has resolved.

Crisis stabilization services that focus, during an initial mobile response period, on a holistic approach through the arrangement of social and physical environments and through consideration of a person with I/DD's expression of their mental health condition, their experience of trauma, and awareness of potential triggers, would effectively inform the type and frequency of services and supports to address the factors contributing to or maintaining the presenting crisis or situation.[49]

SUMMARY

Crisis response is growing across the United States with increasingly broad phone, text, and chat response systems that lead to the need to triage callers who may be in need of further outreach. This might include deploying a mobile crisis response team and/or referring a caller to a crisis stabilization unit. Some individuals will ultimately need psychiatric inpatient hospitalization or acute substance use services. The nuances of the crisis service system continuum are in a period of incredible growth. Most of the crisis response systems have had the issues of persons with mental illness and substance use disorders at the forefront of their planning. It is important, however, to consider the needs of anyone who arrives in a crisis setting. Increasingly, it is recognized that persons with I/DD will also present as having crisis needs, and the systems and providers who support them will need to be prepared. Such individuals may have areas of different abilities along social, communication, and cognitive dimensions. They may present in crisis with other individuals who provide information about them, yet the individuals in crisis will still need to drive their own care. There are countless ways that these matters may play out, both to the benefit of the individual or, if not attended to properly, in a way that could result in trauma, distrust in providers, and poor outcomes. The information set forth earlier aims to help advance the field and individual practices to ensure that persons with I/DD receive equivalent care and treatment with information that helps focus on this population's unique features and needs.

CLINICS CARE POINTS

- A comprehensive diagnostic evaluation for a person with Intellectual and/or Other Developmental Disorders (I/DD) could include an assessment of an individual's cognitive and adaptive functioning, as well as a pre-and-perinatal medical history, a family pedigree, a physical examination, and possible genetic screening or neuroimaging.

- The causes of I/DD are diverse and include genetic and non-genetic causes.

- Co-occurring neurodevelopmental disorders, psychiatric disorders, and medical disorders should be taken into account when caring for a person with I/DD in a crisis setting.

- Communication is critical at every stage of crisis support, especially with an individual with I/DD. Acknowledging and creating processes that provide a person with I/DD with the tools, support, and strategies to effectively communicate and get their needs met should occur at every point of the crisis continuum.

REFERENCES

1. National Guidelines for Behavioral Health Crisis Care Best Practice Toolkit, Substance Abuse and Mental Health Services Administration, Available at: https://www.samhsa.gov/sites/default/files/national-guidelines-for-behavioral-health-crisis-care-02242020.pdf, 2020. Accessed February 26, 2024.
2. National Association of State Mental Health Program Directors, Crisis Services: Addressing Unique Needs of Diverse Populations, Available at: https://www.nasmhpd.org/sites/default/files/2020paper8.pdf, 2020. Accessed February 26, 2024.
3. American Psychiatric Association. Diagnostic and Statistical Manual of mental disorders. 5th edition. Arlington (VA): American Psychiatric Association; 2013.
4. DSM-5 intellectual disability Fact Sheet. American Psychiatric Association, Available at: https://www.psychiatry.org/File%20Library/Psychiatrists/Practice/DSM/APA_DSM-5-Intellectual-Disability.pdf, 2013. Accessed February 26, 2024.
5. Bertelli MO, Cooper S, Salvador-Carulla L. Intelligence and specific cognitive functions in intellectual disability. Curr Opin Psychiatr 2018;31(2):88–95.
6. Lee K., Cascella M., Marwaha R., Intellectual Disability. [Updated 2023 Jun 4]. In: StatPearls [Internet]. Treasure Island (FL): StatPearls Publishing; 2024. Available at: https://www.ncbi.nlm.nih.gov/books/NBK547654/. Accessed June 07, 2024.
7. Julian JN. Intellectual disability. In: Stern TA, Fava M, Wilens TE, editors. Massachusetts General Hospital comprehensive clinical psychiatry. New York: Oxford; 2008. p. 198–204.
8. Totsika V, Liew A, Absoud M, et al. Mental health problems in children with intellectual disability. Lancet Child Adolesc Health 2022;6(6):432–44.
9. Denny L, Coles S, Blitz R. Fetal Alcohol Syndrome and Fetal Alcohol Spectrum Disorders. Am Fam Physician 2017;96(8):515–22.
10. Portes V. Chapter 9-intellectual disability. In: Gallagher A, Bulteau C, Cohen D, editors. Handbook of clinical neurology, 174. Amsterdam, Netherlands: Elsevier; 2020. p. 113–26.

11. Anderson LL, Larson SA, Mapel Lentz S, et al. A systematic review of U.S. studies on the prevalence of intellectual or developmental disabilities since 2000. Intellect Dev Disabil 2019;57(6):421–38.

12. Grantham-McGregor S, Cheung YB, Cueto S, et al. Developmental potential in the first 5 years for children in developing countries. Lancet 2007;369:60–70.

13. Committee to Evaluate the Supplemental Security Income Disability Program for Children with Mental Disorders, Board on the Health of Select Populations, Board on Children, Youth, and Families, Institute of Medicine, Division of Behavioral and Social Sciences and Education, The National Academies of Sciences, Engineering, and Medicine. In: TF Boat, JT Wu, editors. Mental disorders and disabilities among low-income children, Clinical Characteristics of Intellectual Disabilities. Washington, DC: National Academies Press (US); 2015. Available at: https://www.ncbi.nlm.nih.gov/books/NBK332877/.

14. Boyle CA, Boulet S, Schieve LA, et al. Trends in the prevalence of developmental disabilities in U.S. children 1997-2008. Pediatrics 2011;127(6):1034–42.

15. Munir KM. The co-occurrence of mental disorders in children and adolescents with intellectual disability/intellectual developmental disorder. Curr Opin Psychiatr 2016;29(2):95–102.

16. Harris JC. Intellectual disability: understanding its development, causes, classification, evaluation, and treatment. New York: Oxford University Press; 2006.

17. Bouras N, Holt G. Psychiatric and behavioural disorders in developmental disabilities and mental retardation. Cambridge (United Kingdom): Cambridge University Press; 2007.

18. Fletcher RJ, Loschen E, Stavrakaki C, et al, editors. Diagnostic manual-intellectual disability: a textbook of diagnosis of mental disorders in persons with intellectual disability. Kingston, NY: NADD Press; 2007.

19. Tonnsen BL, Boan AD, Bradley CC, et al. Prevalence of autism spectrum disorders among children with intellectual disability. Am J Intellect Dev Disabil 2016;121:487–500.

20. Buckley N, Glasson EJ, Chen W, et al. Prevalence estimates of mental health problems in children and adolescents with intellectual disability: a systematic review and meta-analysis. Aust N Z J Psychiatr 2020;54:970–84.

21. Carroll Chapman SL, Wu LT. Substance abuse among individuals with intellectual disabilities. Res Dev Disabil 2012;33(4):1147–56.

22. Lin E, Balogh R, McGarry C, et al. Substance-related and addictive disorders among adults with intellectual and developmental disabilities (I/DD): an Ontario population cohort study. BMJ Open 2016;6(9):e011638.

23. Devinsky O, Asato M, Camfield P, et al. Delivery of epilepsy care to adults with intellectual and developmental disabilities. Neurology 2015;85(17):1512–21.

24. Seto K, Lloyd M, Chan V, et al. Traumatic Brain Injury Incidence in Adults with Intellectual and Developmental Disabilities. Can J Neurol Sci 2021;48(3):392–9.

25. Slayter EM, Garnick DW, Kubisiak JM, et al. Injury prevalence among children and adolescents with mental retardation. Ment Retard 2006;44(3):212–23.

26. Cox CR, Clemson L, Stancliffe RJ, et al. Incidence of and risk factors for falls among adults with an intellectual disability. J Intellect Disabil Res 2010;54(12):1045–57.

27. Finlayson J, Morrison J, Jackson A, et al. Injuries, falls and accidents among adults with intellectual disabilities: prospective cohort study. J Intellect Disabil Res 2010;54(11):956–80.

28. Hepburn S., Mary sowers on getting rid of policy relics and ensuring 988 works for people with I/DD. CrisisTalk, Available at: https://talk.crisisnow.com/mary-

sowers-on-getting-rid-of-policy-relics-and-ensuring-988-works-for-people-with-idd/, 2022. Accessed June 7, 2024.

29. Hallyburton A. Diagnostic overshadowing: An evolutionary concept analysis on the misattribution of physical symptoms to pre-existing psychological illnesses. Int J Ment Health Nurs 2022;31(6):1360–72.

30. McEntee MK. Accessibility of Mental Health Services and Crisis Intervention to the Deaf. Am Ann Deaf 1993;138:26–30.

31. Diagnostic Manual-Intellectual Disability: A Clinical Guide for Diagnosis (DM-ID-2). Kingston, NY: Press; 2018.

32. Lineberry S, Bogenschutz M, Broda M, et al. Co-Occurring Mental Illness and Behavioral Support Needs in Adults with Intellectual and Developmental Disabilities. Community Ment Health J 2023;59(6):1119–28.

33. Kalb LG, DiBella F, Jang YS, et al. Mental Health Crisis Screening in Youth with Autism Spectrum Disorder [published online ahead of print, 2022 Sep 21]. J Clin Child Adolesc Psychol 2022;1–9.

34. Giarelli E, Nocera R, Turchi R, et al. Sensory stimuli as obstacles to emergency care for children with autism spectrum disorder. Adv Emerg Nurs J 2014;36(2): 145–63.

35. Pinals DA, Hovermale L, Mauch D, et al. The Vital Role of Specialized Approaches: Persons with Intellectual and Developmental Disabilities in the Mental Health System, August 2017. National Association of State Mental Health Program Directors, Center for Mental Health Services, and Substance Abuse and Mental Health Services Administration of the Department of Health and Human Services.

36. Kalb LG, Stuart EA, Vasa RA. Characteristics of psychiatric emergency department use among privately insured adolescents with autism spectrum disorder. Autism 2019;23:566–73.

37. Pinals DA, Fuller DA. Beyond beds: the vital role of a full continuum of psychiatric care. National Association of State Mental Health Program Directors; 2017.

38. Tint A, Lunsky Y. Individual, social and contextual factors associated with psychiatric care outcomes among patients with intellectual disabilities in the emergency department: Psychiatric care in the ED. J Intellect Disabil Res 2015;59:999–1009.

39. McNally P, Taggart L, Shevlin M. Trauma Experiences of People with an Intellectual Disability and their Implications: A Scoping Review. J Appl Res Intellect Disabil 2021;34:927–49.

40. Lunsky Y, Balogh R, Cairney J. Predictors of emergency department visits by persons with intellectual disability experiencing a psychiatric crisis. Psychiatr Serv 2012;63:287–90.

41. Hedman LC, Petrila J, Fisher WH, et al. State Laws on Emergency Holds for Mental Health Stabilization. Psychiatr Serv 2016;67(5):529–35.

42. Americans With Disabilities Act of 1990, 42 U.S.C. § 12101 et seq. (1990).

43. Olmstead v. L.C., 527 U.S. 581; 119 S. Ct. 2176.

44. Administration for Community Living (ACL), HCBS settings rule, Available at: https://acl.gov/programs/hcbs-settings-rule#:~:text=The%20Home%20and%20Community%20Based,in%20the%20most%20integrated%20setting. Accessed February 26, 2024.

45. Heller v. Doe, 509 U.S. 312 (1993).

46. CommunicationFIRST's Style Guide. The words we use, Available at: https://communicationfirst.org/wp-content/uploads/2023/07/C1st-The-Words-We-Use-Style-Guide-v1-July-2023.pdf, 2023. Accessed February 26, 2024.

47. Downey, Jan. The Impact of Anxiety on Communication. Organization for Autism Research, Available at: https://researchautism.org/oaracle-newsletter/the-impact-of-anxiety-on-communication/, 2017. Accessed February 26, 2024.

48. Boardman L, Bernal J, Hollins S. Communicating with people with intellectual disabilities: A guide for general psychiatrists. Adv Psychiatr Treat 2014;20(1):27–36.

49. Schober M, Harburger DS, Sulzbach D, et al. A safe place to be: crisis stabilization services and other supports for children and youth. Technical assistance collaborative paper No. 4. Alexandria (VA): National Association of State Mental Health Program Directors; 2022.

50. Saxon V, Mukherjee D, Thomas D. (2018) Behavioral Health Crisis Stabilization Centers: A New Normal. J Ment Health Clin Psychol 2018;2(3):23–6.

51. National Guidelines for Behavioral Health Crisis Care - Best Practice Toolkit Executive Summary. Substance Abuse and Mental Health Services Administration, Available at: https://www.samhsa.gov/sites/default/files/national-guidelines-for-behavioral-health-crisis-services-executive-summary-02242020.pdf. Accessed February 26, 2024.

52. Pinals DA, Edwards ML. Crisis services: addressing unique needs of diverse populations. Technical assistance collaborative paper No. 8. Alexandria (VA): National Association of State Mental Health Program Directors; 2020.

53. Sugai G, Horner R, Dunlap G, et al. Applying Positive Behavior Support and Functional Behavioral Assessment in Schools. J Posit Behav Interv 2000;2: 131–43.

Policy, Design, and Critical Reflections on Behavioral Health Crisis Services for People Experiencing Homelessness

Samuel W. Jackson, MD[a],*, Enrico G. Castillo, MD, MS[b],
Keris Jän Myrick, MBA, MS[c], Matthew L. Goldman, MD, MS[d]

KEYWORDS

- Homeless • Mental health • Behavioral health • Crisis • Policy

KEY POINTS

- The goal for homeless crisis services cannot be to create the most mentally healthy unhoused population, but rather to address this population's health and social needs, including housing.
- Ideal homeless crisis systems should safeguard against criminalization and displacement, incorporate health equity considerations, and prioritize housing interventions and housing partnerships into every aspect of the system.
- These values must be built into the accountability and financing framework, operationalized in the crisis continuum components, expected as a part of the basic clinical best practices, and tracked for ongoing quality improvement.

INTRODUCTION

While people with serious mental illness (SMI) and substances use disorders (SUDs) are overly represented among people experiencing homelessness (PEH),[1-3] the majority of PEH at any given time do not have an SMI or SUD.[1,2] Drug use, mental illness, and even poverty fail to account for the regional variation in homelessness; instead, lack of affordable housing is in fact the single leading cause.[4] While this report will outline the importance of developing crisis services for PEH, it is essential to state

[a] Department of Psychiatry, SUNY Downstate Health Sciences University, 450 Clarkson Avenue, Brooklyn, NY 11203, USA; [b] Department of Psychiatry, Center for Social Medicine, Jane and Terry Semel Institute for Neuroscience and Human Behavior, David Geffen School of Medicine, UCLA, 760 Westwood Plaza, Semel B7-435, Los Angeles, CA 90095, USA; [c] Inseparable, 409 7th Street N.W. Suite 350 Washington, DC 20004, USA; [d] Department of Psychiatry and Behavioral Sciences, University of Washington, King County Department of Community and Human Resources, 401 5th Avenue, Seattle, WA 98104, USA
* Corresponding author. 392 Street, Marks Avenue Apartment 5C, Brooklyn, NY 11238, USA
E-mail address: samuel.jackson@downstate.edu

Psychiatr Clin N Am 47 (2024) 577–593
https://doi.org/10.1016/j.psc.2024.04.006
0193-953X/24/© 2024 Elsevier Inc. All rights reserved.

psych.theclinics.com

up front that mental illness is not synonymous with homelessness, and the solution to America's homelessness crisis is not more mental health services—it is affordable housing.[4]

Nevertheless, disabilities related to SMI and SUD are significant causes and consequences of homelessness, particularly for unsheltered (ie, living in places not typically designed or used for human habitation such as cars, abandoned buildings, and sidewalks) and chronically homeless individuals.[2,3] Approximately 30% of people experiencing chronic homelessness have an SMI and about two-thirds have a primary SUD, although these estimates range widely.[1–3] With leading causes of death being drug overdose, cardiovascular disease, and cancer as well as having high rates of homicide and suicide, people living in chronic homelessness die up to 25 years earlier than the general population.[5–7] While other prioritized subgroups of PEH have been decreasing—for example, Veteran homelessness has declined 55% since 2010 mostly due to Housing First interventions that prioritize giving permanent supportive housing without preconditions of sobriety or treatment[7]—between 2020 and 2022 unsheltered homelessness increased by 3% and chronic homelessness increased by 16%.[8] Despite decades of research defining cost-effective and compassionate solutions, namely permanent supportive housing,[9–11] many American cities continue to make policy decisions that drive more and more people with mental illness to live in the streets.

When worsening housing instability, substance use, and mental health symptoms lead PEH with SMI or SUD to have more frequent behavioral health crises,[12,13] these often occur in public where the mental health crisis itself or the act of refusing an intervention becomes treated as a crime (eg, disorderly conduct). A well-intentioned bystander calling for help for a person in apparent distress often triggers an armed law enforcement response, leading to an ineffective, costly, and even deadly outcome. With police being the default first responders, individuals in behavioral health crisis account for a quarter of police shootings and more than two million jail bookings each year.[14] Black Americans with mental illness are nearly 10 times more likely to be killed by police than non-Hispanic whites,[15,16] and homelessness further compounds these deadly odds.

Given the high level of needs and ongoing crises in this complex subpopulation of PEH, frequent engagements with first responders and service providers lead them to become "Familiar Faces" within the crisis continuum without being able to engage with the meaningful care that they deserve.[17,18] Whether they were involuntarily admitted to an inpatient psychiatric unit, incapacitated from an overdose in an emergency department, or incarcerated for disorderly conduct, these traumatic interactions with public systems lead to further isolation, entrench experiences of despair and distrust, and narrow the window for change and engagement. Considering the extent of trauma and the sense of rejection both from and toward other components of the crisis continuum, PEH in crisis experience a real lack of meaningful opportunity in improving their immediate situation as well as receiving care. Often lacking a home to sleep in, they also lack a metaphorical home within the crisis continuum.

Fortunately, solutions do exist. With bipartisan political and societal support, there has never been a more opportune time to expand crisis services in general and to implement specific crisis services for PEH.[19,20] Whether a behavioral health crisis system is already firmly established in a community, or a community leader or advocate is thinking about starting one, the roadmap to achieving an ideal crisis system for PEH includes the same principal pathway.[21,22] This article begins with a discussion about structural vulnerability and health equity considerations for behavioral health homeless crisis systems and then presents 3 design elements that we believe are critical for these services: (1) accountability and finance, (2) service continuum and capacities, and (3) clinical best practices. The goal of this article is to provide hope and guidance to communities in the implementation of programs to divert this vulnerable population away from jail and ineffective emergency room visits toward the housing and care that they deserve.

STRUCTURAL VULNERABILITY AND HOMELESS CRISIS SERVICES

Compared to other behavioral health crisis services described in this issue, homeless crisis services have 2 unique qualities that demand consideration. The first is the extreme level of "structural vulnerability"[23] that PEH experience, especially women,[24] lesbian, gay, bisexual, transgender, and queer populations,[25] racially and ethnically minoritized populations,[26] and those experiencing unsheltered homelessness. This high structural vulnerability requires intentional safeguards be in place for homeless crisis services and that such services critically reflect on their relationships with law enforcement and the displacement of encampments (**Box 1**). The second is that homeless crisis services are defined by an unmet social need, specifically housing, which is critical to the goals, design, and implementation of these teams.

Much has been written about the structural vulnerability of PEH.[27–29] With respect to contacts with the criminal justice system, a 2019 study in Los Angeles, California showed that PEH who are unsheltered reported 10 times as many police contacts on average in the previous six months and were nine times as likely to report spending at least one night in jail compared to PEH who were sheltered.[30] Public services and systems in cities and states across the United States contribute to this vulnerability in the ways they interact with this population, especially in the enforcement of laws that police public spaces and criminalize homelessness. States such as Missouri[31] and Tennessee[32] have outlawed PEH from sleeping on state-owned land. Anticamping laws and zones criminalize sleeping, the storage of property, tents, and recreational vehicles in many public spaces, targeting PEH.

For the minority of PEH who have mental illness, this structural vulnerability is even more pronounced. Law professor Jamelia Morgan has written how laws that police public spaces, such as disorderly conduct laws, reinforce saneism against individuals with mental illness through criminalization. She writes, "...disorderly conduct laws tend to criminalize actions that would not be criminal if done in a private place. For example, individuals in mental crises have been charged with disorderly conduct for behaviors that are likely public manifestations of their psychiatric disabilities."[33] Violations can lead to arrests and incarceration.[32] Fines and missed court dates can also lead to arrest warrants and incarceration when PEH cannot afford to pay or miss an appointment.[33]

In addition to criminalization, another vulnerability experienced by PEH is the displacement of individuals and their belongings by law enforcement and other public agencies via sweeps, or the clearing of encampments. Such sweeps move PEH from one part of the city to another, which can lead to loss of property including identification cards and medications, disconnect people from social supports, and disrupt health care and social service use by making it difficult to locate individuals. Research has shown that such sweeps decrease the visible signs of homelessness, but do not lead to PEH achieving permanent housing with a fraction of those displaced even receiving temporary shelter.[34–36]

To be clear, homeless crisis services have the potential to benefit PEH by building caring and trusting relationships and by facilitating referrals to specialized behavioral health treatment, social services, and permanent supportive housing. Homeless crisis

Box 1
Considerations for behavioral health services to acknowledge and address the structural vulnerability experienced by people experiencing homelessness

- Housing: Homeless crisis services must not exist to solely provide behavioral health services but must aim to help individuals achieve permanent supportive housing. Intentional, detailed policies, practices, procedures, and partnerships must be in place to address individuals' housing needs, either directly via access to permanent supportive housing that has been set aside for homeless crisis teams or indirectly through partnerships with local government, private landlords, and community-based housing organizations. Homeless crisis teams should develop formal and informal partnerships with local agencies, organizations, and landlords to increase the permanent supportive housing stock for PEH who receive crisis services. Team members should engage in legislative, media, and other forms of advocacy to increase the availability and accessibility of permanent supportive housing.

- Relationship to Law Enforcement: Homeless crisis services should not in any way further the criminalization of homelessness (eg, arrests, incarceration, fines, warrants), either intentionally or unintentionally. For this reason, we do not recommend that law enforcement be members of homeless crisis teams by default. Non-law enforcement teams should respond to the vast majority of crises involving PEH. When it is necessary that law enforcement co-responds with crisis services (eg, for incidents involving a weapon or active violence), it is the role of crisis teams to protect PEH from criminalization.[15] Additionally, crisis facilities (ie, emergency departments, crisis stabilization centers, comprehensive psychiatric emergency programs) should not call police when discharging a PEH who does not want to leave the facility, as this unnecessarily increases points of contact between the individual and police.

- Protections from Criminalization: Non-law enforcement homeless crisis services should develop memorandums of understanding, policies, and practices to be the preferred response team for behavioral health crises involving PEH. Homeless crisis teams should develop explicit memorandums of understanding with local law enforcement to prevent the inadvertent criminalization of PEH for events that occur in relation to crisis responses, including the prevention of fines/arrest of PEH for minor infractions and misdemeanor agitation/violence.

- Community Partnerships and Involvement of PEH: Homeless crisis services should involve people with lived experience including peer support specialists as team members and as codevelopers of policies, practices, procedures, and trainings. Homeless crisis services should partner with PEH and with local community-based organizations that advocate for and serve this population. Involvement of these partners is particularly important in the codevelopment of policies that safeguard against criminalization and displacement.

- Displacement: Homeless crisis services must be critical about how their actions may intentionally or unintentionally lead to the displacement of PEH (eg, involuntary hospitalization). In cases when crisis involvement leads to or enables displacement (eg, encampment sweeps), homeless crisis teams must be active in ensuring the short- and long-term welfare of PEH who are displaced, especially in connecting displaced PEH to local pathways to permanent housing. Homeless crisis program leadership must also be active at the policy level, ensuring that their locales follow the guidance of the US Interagency Council on Homelessness's "Seven Principles for Addressing Encampments," which cautions against criminalization of PEH and emphasizes pathways to permanent housing and supports.[70]

- Data: Homeless crisis services must collect data on the short- and long-term outcomes of PEH that they serve and participate in integrated data systems that store administrative data from multiple agencies/departments. Differences among definitions of homelessness across systems must be reconciled in order to allow for consistent and reliable data gathering. These data must include process,[71] balance, and outcome measures in behavioral health, criminal legal, and housing domains. Teams, either through data they collect or via their participation in integrated data systems, must be able to track how many individuals obtain permanent supportive housing after the receipt of crisis services. Analyses should also stratify measures by demographic variables such as race/ethnicity to identify and reduce disparities.

services can also work to decriminalize behavioral health crises by decoupling these incidents from responses by law enforcement.[37] Safeguards are critical to ensure that homeless crisis services will truly benefit PEH and prevent inadvertent harms via criminalization and displacement. Homeless crisis services must be critical about their relationships with law enforcement and their potential complicity with criminalization of homelessness. Displacements and sweeps of PEH without clear paths to services and permanent supportive housing must be avoided due to their traumatizing effects and deleterious consequences to individuals' well-being and connections with services and supports. Further, homeless crisis services must be aware of the potential to inadvertently fuel public misinformation and stigma, for example, fueling the misconception that homelessness and mental illness are synonymous or that mental health treatment alone is the solution to homelessness.

However, public services do not necessarily address these vulnerabilities experienced by PEH and can even exacerbate them. In one example from 2019, the city of San Clemente in California banned camping in public places except for a city-supervised camping site. Present onsite were city homeless outreach workers and county health care officials. The city funneled 70 PEH and their belongings into the site, which had no running water or electricity. Shortly after, the city asked individuals at the campsite to leave temporarily so the city could conduct a routine cleanup. When individuals tried to re-enter, city officials demanded they furnish proof of San Clemente residency, barring all but 23 individuals from the campsite and their belongings.[38] This is an example of city laws and public services working in harmony to worsen inequities for PEH.

The same can be true for homeless crisis services; their existence is not a guarantee of benefit for PEH. Because of their proximity to law enforcement and individuals' behaviors (manifestations of mental illness and intoxication) that can be considered crimes (eg, disorderly conduct), homeless crisis services have the potential to be complicit with efforts to criminalize, displace, and harm PEH, rather than addressing their behavioral health or housing needs. Some homeless crisis teams co-respond with law enforcement or even include police officers as members of the team. While these arrangements may be in place to ostensibly protect crisis team members, they can inadvertently place PEH at risk for arrest and criminalization, as law enforcement can exercise "police discretion"[39] to make choices among courses of action including the arrest of individuals in crisis. Calls for homeless crisis services may also originate from individuals in a community who want to quiet or displace PEH from the area. Involuntary hospitalizations, which may be an outcome of homeless crisis services, may clear the way for encampment sweeps, worsening displacements, loss of belongings, and disconnection from social supports and services.

Most importantly, it is imperative for homeless crisis services to understand that it is not enough to provide mental health treatment. The goal for homeless crisis services cannot be to create the most mentally healthy unhoused population. For those PEH with behavioral health needs, it is essential to address their social determinants of health, including housing, to truly address the root causes of their crises. Homeless crisis services should plan to address housing needs, either directly via access to permanent supportive housing or indirectly through robust partnerships with local government, private landlords, and community-based housing organizations. In most locales where adequate permanent supportive housing is not readily available, partnering with organizations that provide homeless maintenance services (ie, aid while homeless including food, water, transportation, and temporary housing such as nighttime shelters or transitional housing) and homeless amelioration services (ie, direct help in getting permanent supportive housing, vocational rehabilitation, and legal aid services) should be part of discharge planning with other interventions in place to maximize success such as warm handoffs, peer support, case management follow-up, and availability of crisis residential type levels of care that can provide a stable environment for continued stabilization. Additionally, homeless crisis services should incorporate community education and advocacy into their activities to address community-level resource deficits. Homeless crisis service providers can share de-identified clinical experiences with policymakers, write op-eds, collaborate with PEH to empower them to share their lived experiences in advocacy venues, or work in other ways to address the structural inequities and system barriers that PEH face. Homeless crisis services should also implement data systems that connect health records with housing databases to track permanent housing, housing retention, law enforcement contacts, arrests, and incarceration for individuals they serve.[40] **Box 1** summarizes some considerations for homeless crisis services.

OVERVIEW OF THE IDEAL CRISIS SYSTEM DESIGN

The remainder of this article outlines how the considerations in **Box 1**, namely addressing the structural vulnerability and housing needs of PEH in crisis, can be built into the ideal crisis system. A brief overview of The Roadmap to the Ideal Crisis System report and its three interacting design elements are provided as a frame for how each element can be tailored to ideally serve PEH in crisis, including examples from communities across the country.

The Roadmap to the Ideal Crisis System was created by the Group for the Advancement of Psychiatry and published by the National Council for Mental Wellbeing in 2021 to provide detailed guidance to communities attempting to implement the best possible behavioral health crisis system for their populations. A companion report, published by the National Council in 2023, provides metrics for crisis systems to measure their quality of care.[41] The Roadmap's vision is that a community's behavioral health crisis system, such as its emergency medical services system, must be more than a siloed program or collection of services but rather a coordinated system with a governance and accountability structure that ensures needs of people in crisis are met in an effective, timely, and cost-effective manner. To achieve this, The Roadmap describes three interacting design elements of an ideal crisis system: (1) accountability and finance, (2) service continuum and capacities, and (3) clinical best practices.[21] The subsequent sections define each of these three elements and describe how they can be tailored to meet the unique crisis needs of PEH (**Fig. 1**).

TAILORING ACCOUNTABILITY AND FINANCE FOR PEOPLE EXPERIENCING HOMELESSNESS IN CRISIS

The first design element describes the mechanism for how a comprehensive crisis system both finances a continuum of crisis services and ensures the quality of the continuum's performance. An "accountable entity" is a vital part of this mechanism whose function is to hold the responsibility of the system performance and may also provide funding or coordinate multiple funding sources. Accountable entities have various forms and may include a county's behavioral health department or local mental health authority such as in Travis County, Texas, a Medicaid managed care organization such as in Tucson, Arizona, or a formal collaborative structure composed of multiple key system partners as in Douglas County, Kansas.[21,42] The "crisis coordinator," a key leadership position usually within the accountable entity, oversees and continually improves each component of the crisis system and regularly convenes meetings with crisis system partners. Importantly, the accountable entities ensure that the values

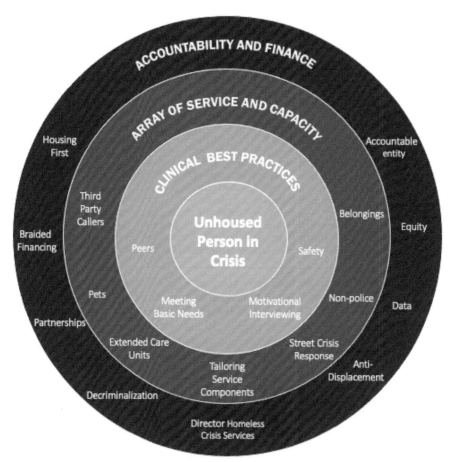

Fig. 1. Depicts the three interacting design elements of an ideal crisis system and how each element can be tailored to address the structural vulnerability and housing needs of PEH in crisis. (*From* the Roadmap to the Ideal Crisis System 2021 Report Published by The National Council.)

of the organization, such as addressing criminalization, displacement, and housing needs of PEH in crisis, are incorporated into all of the organization's processes, including staffing, data collection, quality improvement, and outcomes.[21]

As it pertains to homeless crisis services, the accountable entity, ideally including representation of PEH, must account for the ways in which the current crisis system may exacerbate criminal legal involvement, loss of property, and add barriers to housing, and then be held accountable to address them. Either for a large, single system or a regional collection of smaller crisis systems, funding may be earmarked to ensure adequate, protected time for an additional, administrative leadership role, the "director for homeless crisis services." Working with the crisis coordinator, this person would be responsible for implementing equitable safeguards to PEH in crisis, operating as a communicator, teacher, and system change agent, as well as engaging relevant crisis partners (ie, Department of Homeless Services, permanent supportive housing and transitional housing organizations, social service organizations responsible for benefits, law enforcement, and peer-led advocacy groups) to ensure extant structural vulnerabilities are being addressed.

Health and Hospitals Director of Behavioral Health Homeless Services

Partly in response to problematic outcomes, some large systems, such as New York City's Health and Hospitals, have invested in an analogous type of leadership role. Health and Hospitals, New York City's safety net hospital system, is the single largest provider of care for the approximately 70,000 New Yorkers experiencing homelessness.[43] Serving as both a clinical and administrative leader, the Medical Director of Behavioral Health Homeless Services[44] provides direct patient care, manages multiple extended care units (more details on extended care units discussed later), and hires, trains, and supervises providers in integrated care settings serving PEH only. Additionally, this leader develops and teaches a curriculum to all clinical staff on how to best provide care for this population, works with interagency departments to tailor and create resources for PEH with SMI, and collaborates with various state department stakeholders for further expansion of resources, collaboration, and educational opportunities. The Medical Director of Behavioral Health and Homeless Services has greatly contributed to the expansion of accountable, cost-effective services for PEH with SMI throughout New York City.

Financing a crisis system that ideally services PEH will likely include a mixture of state and local general funds, grant funding, and insurance reimbursement, primarily through Medicaid. Because a significant portion of PEH in crisis will not have insurance (despite many being eligible), a large portion of these services will be paid for by federal block grants, dedicated taxes, and program grants. In Douglas County Kansas, for example, a quarter of a cent sales tax has generated approximately $4.9 million annually to expand behavioral health crisis services as well as supportive housing.[45] Given the inherently collaborative nature of providing these services, funding from behavioral health, social service, housing, and law enforcement agencies may be braided together to provide crisis services.[21,46,47]

The extent to which crisis services can bill Medicaid depends on the state plan as well as managed care reimbursement policies, and many of these policies are currently in flux. In a 2023 survey of state Medicaid programs asking whether they cover three core crisis services (crisis hotlines, mobile crisis units, and crisis stabilization), 33 out of the 45 responding states did not cover all three services, with crisis hotlines being the least likely to be covered.[48] For mobile crisis, reimbursement for engagement efforts is not commonly reimbursed but is particularly important for PEH in crisis as they may only accept services after multiple engagement attempts have been made.[49] Gathering insurance information is difficult during any behavioral health crisis but is particularly challenging for PEH in crisis who may be reluctant to give personal information, provide nonlegal names, or are only identified by bystanders. If basic demographic information is obtained, integrated databases such as Psychiatric Services and Clinical Knowledge Enhancement System[50] and electronic Provider Assisted Claim Entry System[51], in New York State, for example, allow crisis programs to determine which recipients have active Medicaid and retroactively bill for their services.

Despite being eligible, PEH are more likely to have interrupted Medicaid coverage compared to the housed Medicaid population, often due to barriers like not replying to mailed eligibility renewal paperwork.[52] Referred to as "Medicaid churn," this problem has two important consequences for mental health crisis systems: (1) there is evidence that because of the loss of access to preventative health care and social services, Medicaid churn leads to increased use of crisis services, including increased emergency room visits and hospitalizations,[53,54] and (2) without active Medicaid, PEH lose access to a myriad of services addressing their social determinants of health. Programs, such as SOAR (Supplemental Security Income/Social Security Disability Insurance Outreach, Access, and Recovery), Health Homes, and others, eligible through Medicaid, provide case management and peer support to help people sign up for their benefits and make it to follow-up appointments. Additionally, the Centers for Medicare and Medicaid Services (CMS) is starting to experiment with financing health-related social needs, including housing. While historically, Medicaid funds were not permitted to be used to directly pay for housing (ie, rent), CMS is now reframing housing as a social determinant of health. For example, Arizona and New York recently received a Medicaid waiver which allows payments for housing for up to 6 months for individuals transitioning out of places such as congregate settings, homeless shelters, the child welfare system, and others as a way to transition more people out of homelessness.[55,56] Whether it is for direct reimbursement of crisis services or to connect PEH in crisis to housing and other social support, Medicaid is an invaluable part of financing a crisis system for PEH.

Another role that payers can play is looking at their service array and utilization management criteria to ensure that PEH have access to the services they need. We recommend payers use medical necessity criteria such as the Level of Care Utilization System which includes a recovery environment as a domain.[57] For example, PEH might have improved symptoms with a crisis intervention but still need ongoing stabilization in a safe environment such as crisis residential, whereas someone with the same symptoms who is housed could be discharged home. Medical necessity criteria should be able to recognize this distinction.

To incentive housing outcomes, systems may choose to use performance contracting to maximize effectiveness. This would mean that the more housing interventions are made and the more PEH in crisis get placed into housing, the more money crisis teams receive. However, in order to do this, housing needs to be available. The extent to which government-supported housing is needed is related to the housing market (ie, unaffordable housing markets such as San Francisco, Los Angeles, and New York City create a higher need for government-subsidized housing such as permanent supportive housing). Where housing markets are unaffordable, permanent supportive housing is not at scale, and transitional housing (ie, shelters like "safe havens"[58]) is not available, large encampments tend to form.[59] In these communities, advocacy for more affordable housing and permanent supportive housing becomes a vital responsibility of the accountable entity.

CRISIS CONTINUUM CAPACITY AND COMPONENTS FOR PEOPLE EXPERIENCING HOMELESSNESS

The second design element comprises the service continuum and capacities. While a full description of all of the crisis continuum components is outside the scope of this article, depending on the service need and stage of development, a community's crisis continuum may include a crisis hub, 24 hour 988 call center, mobile crisis team, first responders (emergency medical services and crisis intervention team trained police), behavioral health urgent care, crisis facilities including crisis residential, peer respite (especially important if housing is not readily available, peer respite can offer support while PEH in crisis get connected to housing services), 23 hour crisis observation and extended observation, and hospitals including emergency rooms, psychiatric consultation, psychiatric inpatient units, and intensive outpatient services. There should be fluid movement in both directions of the continuum depending on the person's needs[21] and postcrisis follow-up coordinated across all settings. The accountable entity and its partners must continually evaluate the ideal capacity of each crisis service as well as identify priority individuals and communities of greatest need.[21,60] The following are examples of how to think about tailoring specific crisis services to PEH.

Crisis Hotlines

Call centers may develop specific trainings and protocols to prepare for common situations involving PEH in crisis. For example, crisis centers may develop dedicated protocols for third party callers who observe concerning behavior in public spaces (including offering callers the option not to transfer their call to 911 if the only response is police). Third party callers themselves are commonly distressed, so it is important to not only provide appropriate response to the PEH in crisis in these situations but also support and educate the caller. Partnering with local 911 Public Safety Answering Points to identify homelessness-related calls (often there are specific homelessness-related police codes) is important as a way of diverting to nonpolice responses such as mobile crisis or street outreach teams. Importantly, housing needs must be addressed, so for someone identified as experiencing homelessness, housing resources (ideally a warm handoff to a homeless or social service agency) would be offered alongside any behavioral health intervention. Finally, finding PEH in crisis is often difficult, so call centers would ideally set standards for how to collect location information from people who do not have a home address and are calling for help.[61]

Mobile Crisis Teams

Mobile crisis teams ideally include peer specialists with lived experience of homelessness to improve engagement and rapport building with clients.[62] As a means of engagement, mobile crisis teams serving PEH are set up to provide basic needs such as food, water, and housing interventions alongside behavioral health treatment. Mobile crisis teams may develop a direct line to housing and social service agencies or incorporate a representative from those agencies to join when responding to a call for a PEH in crisis. Additionally, mobile crisis teams may find ways to incentivize proactive outreach and engagement activities during down time to high density areas of PEH. As many PEH carry their belongings including pets wherever they go, transport protocols should include best practices for moving personal items and pets to help demonstrate understanding and promote engagement while averting undesirable traumatic outcomes. Many PEH in crisis who have engaged with a mobile crisis team may not need emergency transportation to an emergency department but would benefit from transportation to a shelter or emergency housing, so developing nonemergency transport options and partnerships is another helpful way to tailor these teams to ideally serve PEH.

San Francisco's Street Crisis Response Team

Through a cross-agency collaboration with the Department of Public Health, the San Francisco Fire Department, and community organizations, San Francisco's Street Crisis Response Team is a part of a package of mental health programs for PEH funded by a tax initiative on high-earning businesses in San Francisco. Composed of a paramedic, a behavioral health clinician, and a peer support specialist, this team is dispatched directly from 911 calls coded as having emotional distress and meet people as an alternative to police response. The program aims to avoid unnecessary use of police and costly hospital stays and to address the immediate needs of PEH in the field. They operate 24/7, 365 days a year, have the ability to transport clients to services such as treatment and housing and refer clients to follow-up care and support. Most Street Crisis Response Team engagements are in the areas with the highest density of PEH in San Francisco, confirmation that they are reaching their intended population, and while they are not always able to collect race and ethnicity data, they strive to do so in an effort to emphasize equity as an outcome and quality improvement standard. Their response times are around 17 minutes, and most encounters are resolved in the field with only 6% requiring involuntary removal.[63]

Crisis Receiving and Stabilization Facilities

Similar to mobile crisis teams, crisis stabilization facilities ideally incorporate peer specialists with lived experience of homelessness into the treatment teams. They may provide additional basic needs such as accommodations for secured belongings, showers, laundry, and physical health treatment such as wound care to increase the likelihood of engagement. Also, crisis stabilization spaces may consider creating a "pull model" by colocating crisis facilities with drop-in social services that may be able to complete psychosocial and psychiatric evaluations for housing, ideally embedding housing access within receiving facilities that frequently serve PEH as a Housing First approach.[61]

Subacute Settings: New York City's Extended Care Units

- After being acutely stabilized on an inpatient psychiatric unit, the extended care unit serves as a voluntary, subacute setting where patients experiencing homelessness with SMI can stay up to 120 days. Patients receive rehabilitation through social learning, which, in addition to medication management (including clozapine and electroconvulsive therapy) and psychotherapy, highlights the role of community-based learning (therapeutic groups) and positive behavioral reinforcement (rewards for prosocial behaviors such as doing their laundry or curating a display of artwork) to maneuver through challenges, stressors, and other potentially anxiety provoking situations. Staff, which include peer support specialists, may accompany patients for trips to the grocery store or the subway to practice re-acclimating to living and thriving in the community.[64] Extended care units also provide intensive case management to address social determinants of health including housing, benefits and entitlements, and linkage to proper support in the community including to assertive community treatment[65], intensive mobile treatment[66] as well as medical respite and permanent supportive housing.[64]

- Over a three year period from 2020 to 2023, Bellevue's extended care unit has treated over 200 patients with SMI, most of whom were currently or previously chronically street homeless. Extended care units significantly increase the number of people housed and dramatically reduce emergency room and inpatient utilization post-extended care unit stay. As a cost-effective model, these units are being created in other safety net hospitals across New York City and may be viewed as a model for high intensity services that prioritizes housing and rehabilitation.[64]

IDEAL CLINICAL BEST PRACTICES FOR PEOPLE EXPERIENCING HOMELESSNESS IN CRISIS

The third and final design element identifies the clinical best practices needed to serve PEH in crisis. Using the system's values, such as providing equitable care and safeguarding against criminalization and displacement and using evidence-based interventions, the accountable entity must ensure all staff adopt and adhere to a set of best practice guidelines. These guidelines are incorporated into hiring, training, and ongoing supervision standards, detail what skills each crisis staff member must have, and inform how people in crisis are engaged, assessed, and what treatment interventions are offered in addition to what data get collected. These value-based clinical standards define the expected system performance, and lack of adherence triggers a quality oversight and review process mandatory for staff and services when clinical care does not meet core competency standards.[21]

Three clinical best practices, which are not necessarily unique to crisis care for PEH, are ideally emphasized when serving PEH in crisis: (1) meet basic needs (including food, housing, and safety), (2) incorporate peers, and (3) use motivational interviewing. Providing water, food, housing solutions whether through partnership referrals or incorporation of additional social service team members, and valuing safety, specifically respecting personal space, belongings, and practices that decrease the risk of displacement and unnecessary police involvement not only reflect ideal values but also are aligned with evidence-based practices. Studies find that when staff show that they "really care" by addressing basic needs first, have an "intent to listen," and uphold the person's dignity by respecting their space and belongings, they are better able to engage PEH in treatment.[67,68] Thus, providing basic needs such as housing alongside mental health or addiction treatment as a means of engagement should be a standard approach to PEH in crisis in all components of the continuum.[14]

Given the stigma and shame of homelessness, peers with similar lived experience are uniquely adept at engagement, promoting recovery, and increasing trust. Two studies, including one randomized controlled trial of peers as navigators for unstably unhoused individuals, showed increased engagement with health care, support services, and housing support as well as significantly reduced mental health concerns and psychological distress, reduced anxiety, decreased rates of injection drug use, increased access to resources, and reduced homelessness at the 12 month intervention period.[60,62] As of 2022, seven states require peer support on mobile crisis teams, and similar requirements are being pursued in 13 additional states in 2023.[48] Peers with lived experience of homelessness are ideally incorporated into every aspect of an ideal crisis system serving PEH.

Motivational interviewing is another person-centered approach toward engagement of individuals expressing ambivalence by aiming to enhance someone's motivation to change.[69] Studies examining motivational interviewing with PEH, including four randomized controlled trials of between two to four sessions of motivational interviewing, have shown a reduction of alcohol, cocaine, amphetamine, and opiate use, increased readiness to reduce or quit other drugs, as well as increased service utilization at one month follow-up.[60] Training on motivational interviewing is available for clinician and nonclinician staff alike, does not have a prescribed length or duration, and should be a clinical best practice for engagement and intervention throughout the crisis continuum.

SUMMARY

PEH in crisis have unique structural vulnerabilities and social needs, most importantly lack of housing. Ideal crisis services for PEH must safeguard against the criminalization and displacement of PEH in crisis, prioritize equity, and provide housing interventions at every stage in the crisis continuum. The accountable entity along with the director of crisis homeless services is responsible for taking these structural vulnerabilities and social needs into account, addressing existing harmful practices, incorporating value-based interventions, and building necessary collaborations with housing services, community members, data systems, and other partners. Each crisis service, such as call centers, mobile crisis, and crisis stabilization centers, ideally serves PEH through engagement by peer specialists, respecting their space and belongings, and providing basic needs alongside mental health services. By outlining how to tailor crisis system financing and accountability, service component and capacity, and clinical best practices, we aim to provide hope and guidance for communities implementing ideal crisis services for PEH. These special considerations may mean the difference between someone getting forcibly relocated or jailed versus getting humanely housed and receiving treatment.

CLINICS CARE POINTS

- Crisis interventions should safeguard against criminalization, loss of belongings and animals, disruption of services and social supports, and displacement.
- Crisis services are opportunities to address not only behavioral health needs but also basic needs, such as providing food, water, safe storage of belongings, housing, and connection to local services.
- The goal is not to create the most mentally healthy unhoused population; crisis services working with PEH should directly address or partner with organizations to mitigate social determinants of health, including housing.

DISCLOSURE

Dr E.G. Castillo has received funding from the National Institute of Mental Health (K23 MH-125201). Other authors have nothing to disclose.

REFERENCES

1. The 2022 Annual Homelessness Assessment Report (AHAR) to Congress. The U.S. Department of Housing and Urban Development. 2022. Available at: https://www.huduser.gov/portal/sites/default/files/pdf/2022-ahar-part-1.pdf.
2. Substance Abuse and Mental Health Services Administration. Current Statistics on the Prevalence and Characteristics of People Experiencing Homelessness in the United States. 2011. Available at: https://www.samhsa.gov/sites/default/files/programs_campaigns/homelessness_programs_resources/hrc-factsheet-current-statistics-prevalence-characteristics-homelessness.pdf. [Accessed 22 August 2020].
3. Toward a New Understanding: The California Statewide Study of People Experiencing Homelessness. Benioff homelessness and housing initiative. San Francisco: University of California; 2023. p. 1–96. Available at: https://homelessness.ucsf.edu/sites/default/files/2023-06/CASPEH_Report_62023.pdf.
4. Colburn G, Aldern CP. Homelessness is a housing problem: how structural factors explain U.S. Patterns. University of California Press; 2022.
5. Funk AM, Greene RN, Dill K, et al. The impact of homelessness on mortality of individuals living in the United States: a systematic review of the literature. J Health Care Poor Underserved 2022;33(1):457–77.
6. Brown RT, Evans JL, Valle K, et al. Factors Associated With Mortality Among Homeless Older Adults in California: The HOPE HOME Study. JAMA Intern Med 2022;182(10):1052.
7. Baggett TP, Hwang SW, O'Connell JJ, et al. Mortality among homeless adults in boston: shifts in causes of death over a 15-Year Period. JAMA Intern Med 2013; 173(3):189.
8. New Data Shows 11% Decline in Veteran Homelessness Since 2020—the Biggest Drop in More Than 5 Years. U.S. Department of Housing and Urban Development. 2022. Available at: https://www.hud.gov/press/press_releases_media_advisories/hud_no_22_225.

9. HUD Releases 2022 Annual Homeless Assessment Report. U.S. Department of Housing and Urban Development. 2022. Available at: https://www.hud.gov/press/press_releases_media_advisories/hud_no_22_253.

10. Raven MC, Niedzwiecki MJ, Kushel M. A randomized trial of permanent supportive housing for chronically homeless persons with high use of publicly funded services. Health Serv Res 2020;55(S2):797–806.

11. Aubry T, Bloch G, Brcic V, et al. Effectiveness of permanent supportive housing and income assistance interventions for homeless individuals in high-income countries: a systematic review. Lancet Public Health 2020;5(6):e342–60.

12. Rog DJ, Marshall T, Dougherty RH, et al. Permanent supportive housing: assessing the evidence. PS 2014;65(3):287–94.

13. Lee KH, Jun JS, Kim YJ, et al. Mental health, substance abuse, and suicide among homeless adults. J Evidence Informed Soc Work 2017;14(4):229–42.

14. Koh KA. Psychiatry on the streets—caring for homeless patients. JAMA Psychiatr 2020;77(5):445–6.

15. Balfour ME, Hahn Stephenson A, Delany-Brumsey A, et al. Cops, clinicians, or both? collaborative approaches to responding to behavioral health emergencies. PS 2022;73(6):658–69.

16. Saleh AZ, Appelbaum PS, Liu X, et al. Deaths of people with mental illness during interactions with law enforcement. Int J Law Psychiatr 2018;58:110–6.

17. Russolillo A, Moniruzzaman A, Parpouchi M, et al. A 10-year retrospective analysis of hospital admissions and length of stay among a cohort of homeless adults in Vancouver, Canada. BMC Health Serv Res 2016;16(1):1–10.

18. North CS, Smith EM. A systematic study of mental health services utilization by homeless men and women. Soc Psychiatr Psychiatr Epidemiol 1993;28(2):77–83.

19. ALL IN: The Federal Strategic Plan to Prevent and End Homelessness. United States Interagency Council on Homelessness. 2022. Available at: https://www.usich.gov/All_In_The_Federal_Strategic_Plan_to_Prevent_and_End_Homelessness.pdf. [Accessed 27 July 2023].

20. Balfour M. Behavioral Health Crisis Care's Carpe Diem Moment. Psychiatric Times. 2022. Available at: https://www.psychiatrictimes.com/view/behavioral-health-crisis-care-s-carpe-diem-moment.

21. Roadmap to the Ideal Crisis System. National Council for Mental Wellbeing. 2021. Available at: https://www.thenationalcouncil.org/wp-content/uploads/2022/02/042721_GAP_CrisisReport.pdf.

22. Jackson S, Minkoff K, LeMelle S. A roadmap for helping people who are homeless and mentally Ill. Psychol Today 2023. Available at: https://www.psychologytoday.com/us/blog/psychiatrys-think-tank/202301/a-roadmap-to-help-people-who-are-homeless-and-mentally-ill.

23. Bourgois P, Holmes SM, Sue K, et al. Structural vulnerability: operationalizing the concept to address health disparities in clinical care. Acad Med 2017;92(3):299–307.

24. Meinbresse M, Brinkley-Rubinstein L, Grassette A, et al. Exploring the experiences of violence among individuals who are homeless using a consumer-led approach. Violence Vict 2014;29(1):122–36.

25. Flatley CA, Hatchimonji DR, Treglia D, et al. Adolescent homelessness: Evaluating victimization risk based on LGBT identity and sleeping location. J Adolesc 2022;94(8):1108–17.

26. Rhee TG, Rosenheck RA. Why are black adults over-represented among individuals who have experienced lifetime homelessness? Oaxaca-Blinder

decomposition analysis of homelessness among US male adults. J Epidemiol Community Health 2020. jech-2020-214305.

27. Desmond M. Evicted: poverty and profit in the American city. First paperback edition. B\D\W\Y Broadway Books; 2017.

28. Perry AM. Know your price: valuing black lives and property in America's black cities. Brookings Institution Press; 2020.

29. Rothstein R. The color of law: a forgotten history of how our government segregated America. First published as a liveright paperback 2018. Liveright Publishing Corporation, a division of W.W. Norton & Company; 2018.

30. Rountree J, Hess N, Austin L. *Health Conditions Among Unsheltered Adults in the U.S.* California Policy Lab. 2019. Available at: https://www.capolicylab.org/wp-content/uploads/2023/02/Health-Conditions-Among-Unsheltered-Adults-in-the-U.S..pdf.

31. Schoenig Elyse. New law makes sleeping, camping on state-owned land illegal and leaves homeless shelters concerned. 5 on your side. 2023. Available at: https://www.ksdk.com/article/news/local/new-law-makes-sleeping-camping-on-state-owned-land-illegal-and-leaves-homeless-shelters-concerned/63-93058191-ddc0-491d-aa14-b47062162330.

32. The Associated Press. Tennessee is about to become the 1st state to make camping on public land a Felony. NPR News; 2022. Available at: https://www.npr.org/2022/05/26/1101434831/public-camping-felony-tennessee-homeless-seek-refuge.

33. Morgan JN. Rethinking disorderly conduct. Calif Law Rev 2021. https://doi.org/10.15779/Z38KD1QM20.

34. Perez R. Homeless encampment sweeps may be draining your city's budget. 2023. Available at: https://housingmatters.urban.org/feature/homeless-encampment-sweeps-may-be-draining-your-citys-budget#:~:text=Sweeps%20reduce%20the%20visibility%20of,homelessness%20while%20straining%20city%20budgets.

35. Roy A, Bennett A, Blake J, et al. (Dis)Placement: The Fight for Housing and Community After Echo Park Lake. UCLA Luskin Institute on Inequality and Democracy. 2022. Available at: https://escholarship.org/uc/item/70r0p7q4.

36. Lander B, Hayes-Chaffe M. Audit of the Department of Homeless Services' Role in the "Cleanups" of Homeless Encampments. 2023. Available at: https://comptroller.nyc.gov/wp-content/uploads/documents/ME23_059A.pdf.

37. Rafla-Yuan E, Chhabra DK, Mensah MO. Decoupling crisis response from policing — a step toward equitable psychiatric emergency services. In: Malina D, editor. N Engl J Med 2021;384(18):1769–73.

38. Ritchie EI. San Clemente clears homeless camp site and requires proof of ties to the city for reentry. Orange Cty Regist (Santa Ana, CA) 2019. Available at: https://www.ocregister.com/2019/08/30/san-clemente-clears-homeless-camp-site-and-requires-proof-of-ties-to-the-city-for-reentry/. [Accessed 27 July 2023].

39. Reed B. Issues and trends in police discretion. Police Chief 1980;47(11):54–9.

40. Rafla-Yuan E. Mobile crisis metrics: moving toward a functional crisis continuum of care. PS 2023;74(7):673.

41. Goldman M, Shoyinka S, Allender Brian, et al. Quality measurement in crisis services. The National Council for Mental Wellbeing; 2023. Available at: https://www.thenationalcouncil.org/wp-content/uploads/2023/01/23.01.13_Quality-Measurement-in-Crisis-Services.pdf. [Accessed 21 January 2024].

42. Jackson S. Evaluation of a pilot learning community. Group Adv Psychiatr 2022. Available at: https://crisisroadmap-prod.s3.amazonaws.com/resources/attach ments/3f9e972f27ed0d7e9e57548aaf409860.pdf.

43. Basic Facts About Homelessness: New York City. Coalition for the Homeless 2023. Available at: https://www.coalitionforthehomeless.org/basic-facts-about-homelessness-new-york-city/#:~:text=In%20December%202022%2C%20there%20were,each%20night%20in%20December%202022.

44. Nzodom C, Herpen R, Hemphill N. VIDEO: Collaboration key to provide behavioral health services for homeless population. 2023. Available at: https://www.healio.com/news/psychiatry/20230622/video-collaboration-key-to-provide-behavioral-health-services-for-homeless-population. [Accessed 3 August 2023].

45. Masenthin. Kansas community mental health centers transitioning to new care model; Bert Nash is in the first phase. The Lawrence Times 2022. Available at: https://lawrencekstimes.com/2022/05/16/ks-cmhcs-new-model/.

46. Grant Programs and Services for Homelessness. Substance abuse and mental health services. 2023. Available at: https://www.samhsa.gov/homelessness-programs-resources/grant-programs-services.

47. Atkeson A. CalAIM: Leveraging Medicaid Managed Care for Housing and Homelessness Support. National Academy For State Health Policy 2022. Available at: https://www.nashp.org/wp-content/uploads/2022/04/CalAIM-Housing_FINAL.pdf.

48. Saunders H, Guth M, Panchal N. Behavioral health crisis response: findings from a survey of state Medicaid programs. KFF; 2023. Available at: https://www.kff.org/medicaid/issue-brief/behavioral-health-crisis-response-findings-from-a-survey-of-state-medicaid-programs/.

49. Olivet J, Bassuk E, Elstad E, et al. Outreach and engagement in homeless services: a review of the literature~!2009-08-18~!2009-09-28~!2010-03-22. TOHSPJ 2010;3(2):53–70.

50. About Psyckes. New York State Office of Mental Health. Available at: https://omh.ny.gov/omhweb/psyckes_medicaid/about/#:~:text=PSYCKES%20stands%20for%20the%20Psychiatric,billing%20claims%20and%20encounter%20data. [Accessed 14 August 2023].

51. What Is EPACES. New York State electronic Medicaid New York System. Available at: https://epaces.emedny.org/help/What_is_ePACES.htm#:~:text=ePACES%20is%20the%20electronic%20Provider,New%20York%20(eMedNY)%20system. [Accessed 14 August 2023].

52. Dapkins I, Blecker SB. Homelessness and Medicaid Churn. Ethn Dis 2021;31(1):89–96.

53. Hall AG, Harman JS, Zhang J. Lapses in Medicaid coverage: impact on cost and utilization among individuals with diabetes enrolled in Medicaid. Med Care 2008;46(12):1219–25.

54. Ji X, Wilk AS, Druss BG, et al. Discontinuity of Medicaid coverage: impact on cost and utilization among adult Medicaid beneficiaries with major depression. Med Care 2017;55(8):735–43.

55. Centers for Medicare & Medicaid Services. HHS Approves Arizona's Medicaid Interventions to Target Health-Related Social Needs. 2022. Available at: https://www.cms.gov/newsroom/press-releases/hhs-approves-arizonas-medicaid-interventions-target-health-related-social-needs. [Accessed 21 January 2024].

56. Centers for Medicare & Medicaid Services. CMS Approves New York's Groundbreaking Section 1115 Demonstration Amendment to Improve Primary Care, Behavioral Health, and Health Equity. 2024. Available at: https://www.cms.gov/newsroom/press-releases/cms-approves-new-yorks-groundbreaking-section-11

15-demonstration-amendment-improve-primary-care. [Accessed 21 January 2024].

57. American Association for Community Psychiatry. Level of Care Utilization Systems for Psychiatric and Addiction Services. Accessed January 21, 2024. Available at: https://www.communitypsychiatry.org/keystone-programs/locus.

58. New Safe Havens in Brooklyn. Breaking Ground. 2017. Available at: https://breakingground.org/news-events/new-safe-havens-in-brooklyn.

59. Swept Away: Reporting on the Encampment Closure Crisis. National Coalition for the Homeless. 2016. Available at: https://nationalhomeless.org/wp-content/uploads/Swept-Away-2016.pdf.

60. Expanding Access to and Use of Behavioral Health Services for People Experiencing Homelessness. Substance Abuse and Mental Health Services 2023. Available at: https://store.samhsa.gov/sites/default/files/pep22-06-02-003.pdf.

61. Experiencing homelessness and crisis. 2022. Available at: https://www.youtube.com/watch?v=PkNsR0W6Mbl.

62. Peer Support Services in Crisis Care. Substance Abuse and Mental Health Services 2022. Available at: https://store.samhsa.gov/sites/default/files/pep22-06-04-001.pdf.

63. Street Crisis Response Team. City & County of San Francisco. Available at: https://sf.gov/street-crisis-response-team. [Accessed 3 August 2023].

64. Innovative New unit for patients with severe mental illness opens at NYC health + hospitals/kings county. NYC Health + Hospitals; 2023. Available at: https://www.nychealthandhospitals.org/pressrelease/innovative-new-unit-for-patients-with-severe-mental-illness-opens-at-nyc-health-hospitals-kings-county/. [Accessed 3 August 2023].

65. Assertive Community Treatment. New York State Office of Mental Health. Available at: https://omh.ny.gov/omhweb/act/. [Accessed 3 August 2023].

66. Intensive Mobile Treatment (IMT) Teams. NYC Mayor's Office of Community Mental Health. 2019. Available at: https://mentalhealth.cityofnewyork.us/program/intensive-mobile-treatment-imt. [Accessed 3 August 2023].

67. Hwang SW, Burns T. Health interventions for people who are homeless. Lancet 2014;384(9953):1541–7.

68. O'Campo P, Kirst M, Schaefer-McDaniel N, et al. Community-Based Services for Homeless Adults Experiencing Concurrent Mental Health and Substance Use Disorders: A Realist Approach to Synthesizing Evidence. J Urban Health 2009; 86(6):965–89.

69. Miller WR, Rollnick S. Motivational interviewing: helping people change. 3rd edition. Guilford Press; 2013.

70. U.S. Interagency Council on Homelesness. 7 Principles for addressing encampments. U.S. Interagency Council on Homelessness; 2022. Available at: https://www.usich.gov/resources/uploads/asset_library/Principles_for_Addressing_Encampments.pdf. [Accessed 25 August 2023].

71. How to Improve: Model for Improvement. Institute for Healthcare Improvement, Available at: https://www.ihi.org/resources/how-to-improve. (Accessed 7 July 2023).

Youth Crisis
The Current State and Future Directions

Ashley A. Foster, MD[a],*, Michelle Zabel, MSS[b],
Melissa Schober, MPM[b]

KEYWORDS

- Crisis services • Psychiatric emergency services • Mobile crisis teams
- Community mental health services • Pediatric mental health
- Pediatric behavioral health

KEY POINTS

- The number of youth experiencing behavioral health crisis is increasing in the United States.
- Current crisis response systems are often adult-centric and, as such, are not optimally designed to respond to the needs of youth and their families.
- Developing, implementing, studying, and sustaining systems that prioritize maintaining youth in crisis within their home and community are essential.
- Focus on the development of care models that ameliorate racial, ethnic, and other demographic disparities are urgently needed.

INTRODUCTION
The Current State

Behavioral health conditions, including mental health conditions and substance use disorders, are common in youth in the United States (US), with approximately 1 in 5 youth experiencing mental illness every year.[1] Suicide is now the second leading cause of death in youth in the US and worldwide.[2,3] Despite the growing need for pediatric behavioral health care, many counties (47%) do not have access to mental health facilities that provide outpatient treatment to youth, and the number of inpatient psychiatry beds has been declining.[4,5] Additionally, there is a pediatric mental health workforce shortage—there are approximately 8300 practicing child psychiatrists to care for 15 million children with behavioral health conditions.[6,7] Because of the mismatch in need and available resources, 50% to 70% of youth in the US with treatable behavioral health conditions do not receive treatment from a mental health

[a] Department of Emergency Medicine, University of California, San Francisco, 550 16th Street, Box 0649, San Francisco, CA 94143, USA; [b] Innovations Institute, University of Connecticut School of Social Work, 38 Prospect Street, Hartford, CT 06103, USA
* Corresponding author.
E-mail address: Ashley.Foster@ucsf.edu

Psychiatr Clin N Am 47 (2024) 595–611
https://doi.org/10.1016/j.psc.2024.06.001
0193-953X/24/© 2024 Elsevier Inc. All rights reserved, including those for text and data mining, AI training, and similar technologies.

psych.theclinics.com

professional.[8] This may carry substantial consequences: one study found US county mental health professional workforce shortage designation was associated with an increased youth suicide rate.[9]

The coronavirus disease 2019 (COVID-19) pandemic has accelerated challenges for youth, who have experienced social isolation as a result of attempts to mitigate the spread of the virus, school disruptions, caregiver illness and loss, and discontinuity of care.[10] As a consequence, there is an increase in the proportion of youth suffering from anxiety and depression.[11] Subsequently, there has been an increase in youth seeking emergency care for behavioral health crises, including in rural areas.[12,13] By 2021, several pediatric health organizations and the US Surgeon General declared a national state of emergency in children's mental health.[14,15]

These factors have contributed to use of the emergency department (ED) as a safety net by youth in behavioral health crisis both before and during the COVID-19 pandemic.[16,17] While in the ED, youth with behavioral health conditions may have limited access to mental health assessment and treatment and experience prolonged length of stays while awaiting inpatient bed availability, which is often referred to as ED boarding.[18,19] Youth experiencing ED boarding may not have access to therapeutic treatment interventions, pediatric-specific resources, or age-appropriate activities.[20,21] ED boarding also results in adverse medication events, delays in care, and ED staff moral distress.[20,22–24] Additionally, there are specific populations who face prolonged ED boarding including Hispanic youth and children with autism spectrum disorder (ASD) or developmental delays.[18,25]

These data emphasize the need to expand a comprehensive, customized crisis continuum for youth, caregivers, and families. The continuum must be rooted in system of care values and principles: family/caregiver-and-youth-driven, home-based and community-based, equitable, culturally humble, linguistically competent, fully accessible, strengths-based and individualized, data-driven, outcome-oriented, and trauma-responsive.[26,27] An ideal system should be collaborative, as a youth in crisis is likely to need engagement from multiple services and supports (eg, primary care, school, home-based and community-based service providers, child welfare, and community-based organizations). This article describes the recommended continuum of care for youth in behavioral health crisis and discusses existing literature as well as disparities to behavioral health care, current knowledge gaps, and opportunities for future study.

POPULATIONS THAT EXPERIENCE BEHAVIORAL HEALTH INEQUITIES

Although the national rise in youth in behavioral health crisis is alarming on its own, youth from historically underserved racial and ethnic groups; those with diverse sexual orientation, gender identity, and expression (SOGIE); those residing in rural areas; and non-Hispanic American Indian or Alaskan native children are disproportionately burdened by suicide.[28,29]

Racism is an organized system by which the dominant group "devalues, disempowers, and differentially allocates desirable societal opportunities and resources to racial groups categorized as inferior."[30] Families and youth experience structural racism in their homes and communities due to lack of access to quality and culturally sensitive care,[31] provider bias, and deficit-focused institutional practices (ie, focused on the problems of an individual or community, rather than its strengths and assets),[32] all of which have harmed youth and families of color and deepen intergenerational and community trauma.

Black children aged 5 to 12 years have suicide rates 2 times higher than those of similarly aged White children.[33] Between 2003 and 2017, the rate of suicide among

Black youth increased each year, with the suicide rate for girls increasing an average of 6.6% each year—more than twice the increase for boys.[34]

Suicide rates for children and youth are higher in rural areas than in urban communities.[35] From 2010 to 2018, the incidence of suicide for youth aged 10 to 19 years increased 1.5 times faster than same-age youth in urban centers.[36,37] Mental health provider shortages, local service accessibility, poor commercial insurance coverage, underinsurance, and access to lethal means are cited in the literature as contributing factors to the disparity.[38]

In 2017, SOGIE-identified youth were 3 times as likely to attempt suicide compared to their heterosexual peers.[29] Researchers have theorized that SOGIE-identified youth are at an increased risk for behavioral health conditions due to hostile social environments,[39] internalized discrimination, parental rejection, lack of access to welcoming providers, and housing instability.[40]

Youth involved with child welfare systems have a high prevalence of behavioral health conditions associated with suicide and are "significantly more likely than their peers outside the system to engage in suicidal behavior."[41,42] Nearly half of children and young adolescents with completed child welfare investigations had an identified behavioral health concern. Removal from the home is itself a traumatic experience and has been linked to poorer behavioral and physical health outcomes.[43] As young children (aged 1–5 years) are the largest share of children entering care (just under 30% in 2021),[44] mental health providers and crisis response systems must be prepared to serve the needs of the very young and their families.

Over 5 million children in the US have an intellectual or developmental disability (IDD).[45] In 2020, 1 in 36 children was estimated to have ASD with the prevalence and median age of identification varying widely across states.[46] Co-occurring behavioral health conditions are more common in individuals with ASD than the general population.[47] Lack of access to disability-competent care is a significant challenge for many youth and families. Additionally, youth with IDD often face difficulty when transiting to adult systems with some continuing to see pediatric clinicians well into adulthood.[48] Recognizing this, crisis systems must include information about and require training for youth with IDD and ASD to effectively refer for early intervention services, behavioral assessments, home-based and community-based services, and caregiver education and training.[49]

A Recommended Crisis Continuum of Care for Youth

Emerging models for a continuum of crisis services that include community-based services and supports may reduce the need for emergency and inpatient psychiatric care. An ideal system should match the urgency of the youth and caregiver(s) with the ability to respond in-person, 24 hours per day, 7 days per week, anywhere in the US. Given that the developmental, social, and clinical needs of youth are different from adults, youth care models should differ from adult systems in that every effort should be made to keep the child within the home and community for care (**Fig. 1**).[50] The continuum of care should also provide sustained support during the immediate crisis and after crisis intervention, and these supports may continue for up to 6 to 8 weeks.[50,51] Core recommended elements of a comprehensive crisis system include a "no wrong door" system[50,51]: "someone to talk to" (crisis call and text lines), "someone to respond" (mobile response), and "a safe place to be" (home- and community-based stabilization services and acute care services customized for the unique needs of youth, including when an assessment indicates that a youth cannot be safely treated in the home or community).[50,51] "No

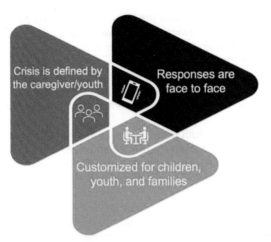

Fig. 1. An ideal youth crisis model. The 3 triangles are a graphical illustration of the essential and inseparable elements of a crisis response model that is designed to meet the unique needs of youth and families beginning with the initial call and continuing through a timely, in-person response. (*Derived from* Schober, M., Harburger, D.S., Sulzbach, D., Zabel, M. (2022). A Safe Place to Be: Crisis Stabilization Services and Other Supports for Children and Youth. Technical Assistance Collaborative Paper No. 4. Alexandria, VA: National Association of State Mental Health Program Directors. https://store.samhsa.gov/sites/default/files/SAMHSA_Digital_Download/nasmhpd-a-safe-place-to-be.pdf.)

wrong door" indicates that all youth and families can receive the services based on self-identified need, regardless of ability to pay or diagnostic condition.[50]

Someone to talk to

Through telephone, texting, or online chat, crisis lines provide emotional support and brief interventions for youth experiencing crisis, with 24 hour availability.[52] Crisis lines may circumvent challenges to accessing traditional mental health services including stigma, uncertainty in where to seek help, and socioeconomic barriers. A 2021 systematic review of studies of youth helplines revealed that much of available data are focused on content analysis of call and text transcripts, which provide information on the types of issues raised by those accessing hotlines.[52] Overall synthesis of youth studies outline the potential positive relationship of helplines in supporting youths with a variety of psychosocial concerns, including suicidality.[52] Future study on long-term effectiveness of hotline services among children of differing ages, with or without ancillary crisis services, are needed.

In 2020, the US Congress passed the National Suicide Hotline Designation Act, which established the 988 Suicide and Crisis Lifeline, building on an existing network of 200 call centers across the US. The legislation delegated responsibility for implementing 988 to individual states, including infrastructure development, hiring and training staff, and integrating 988 with existing emergency service lines. As states develop 988, attention must be given to the specific customizations necessary to support youth callers and their caregivers. Each center must have the technological infrastructure to collect and share information about service recipients.[53] Furthermore, call centers must establish minimum training standards for call triage that include specialized training in child and adolescent development (expected developmental milestones, typical challenging behaviors of childhood and adolescence, behaviors that indicate more significant behavioral health concerns) as well as how to support the family during the acute crisis period.[54] Current barriers to offering robust crisis continuum services through 988 include limited funding, workforce shortages, and geographic constraints.[55] For example, as of June 2023, only 26 states have appropriated 988 funding or authorized a 988 telecom fee to be collected to support 988 services.[56]

Text messaging has now become a dominant form of communication among youths, who report that texting is a more private and comfortable way of communicating than calling or talking face-to-face and can provide help in the moment of symptoms.[57,58] Data from the Lifeline Crisis Chat network reveal that out of 39,911 chats connected to a chat counselor and included in the analysis, nearly 40% were children aged less than 17 years and 70% were aged 24 years or less.[59] Surveys from the study showed that chatters were significantly less distressed by the end of chat intervention compared to at the beginning of the chat.[59] Another study that described the population of individuals who utilize crisis text support found nearly 30% of chatters aged 24 years or less received help from a crisis text line only.[60] This finding identifies that crisis text may be the only point of contact for youth in behavioral health distress and reinforces the guidance that an increased development of crisis services integration is important.[50] Additional study around best practices for text communication with children and impact of text communication on long-term patient outcomes will ensure crisis texting is a safe and effective platform for youth.

In an optimally envisioned fully comprehensive call center system, crisis line clinicians can respond to intensive crisis referrals by dispatching Global Positioning System-enabled mobile crisis teams, have the capabilities to schedule outpatient appointments, and when needed, visualize openings at crisis stabilization units (CSUs) capable of serving children and youth populations, as well as psychiatric inpatient bed availability, through an online system.[53] However, additional supports and resources will be required to achieve this goal including growing mobile response capacity, enhancing outpatient behavioral health capacity, and increasing transparency around pediatric CSU and psychiatric inpatient bed availability within a state. Currently, only 17 states have bed tracking systems, with 5 of these states providing direct public access to bed-tracking information.[61] An additional challenge is that in many parts of the US, law enforcement and emergency medical services (EMS) are accessed as first responders to youth in behavioral health crisis.[50] Enhancing resources and availability of crisis response would allow 911 to divert appropriate calls to 988 crisis call centers, which could facilitate EMS to be used specifically for youth in imminent danger or for youth with concomitant medical symptoms who require ED evaluation.[50]

Someone to respond

Mobile crisis teams (MCTs) are one to two-person units that consist of trained clinicians, behavioral health technicians, and/or peer support providers. These teams meet youth and caregivers/families within the community, including at home, in school, on the street, at CSUs, and within the ED, upon caller request.[50,62,63] MCTs de-escalate crises, assess immediate basic needs of the youth and their caregivers, conduct trauma-responsive and individualized screening and assessments, facilitate connection to natural supports, and engage the youth and families in initial care and referral planning, as needed.[51] In a developed mobile response model, there are also stabilization services provided up to 8 weeks after the initial assessment.[50] These stabilization services can link individuals with community-based supports such as caregiver education, youth development and recreational programs, and clinical and school-based services. Additionally, in a comprehensive crisis system, if the

MCT's assessment of the youth indicates that care cannot be met in a community-based setting, a state or locality's bed registry can be used to access a CSU or inpatient bed.

Currently available literature about MCT response to youth in crisis is promising. One study shows that youth served by MCTs have lower odds of subsequent behavioral health ED visits compared to youth in a comparison sample,[64] and another study showed only 3.2% of youth who received services from MCT received inpatient care within 30 days of that encounter.[65] Additionally, data from a program in Massachusetts that included youth encounters reported that as MCT programs were implemented, a lower proportion of encounters occurred in the ED over time with correspondingly more frequent responses occurring within the community.[66]

Although staffing models for MCTs have not yet been studied, the Centers for Medicare & Medicaid Services provided guidance on MCTs and recommended "incorporating trained peers who have lived experience in recovery from mental illness and/or substance use disorders and formal training within the MCT; responding without law enforcement accompaniment, unless special circumstances warrant inclusions, in order to support justice system diversion."[67] Peer support for youth with behavioral health conditions has been linked to reductions in disparities related to outpatient service access.[68] Additionally, youth participating in peer support and engagement have reported an increased hope for the future and sense of belonging when participating in groups cofacilitated by peers and clinicians.[69] Contrastingly, the presence of police during a behavioral health crisis may exacerbate anxiety and trauma faced by youth, particularly for individuals and families of color.[70] Additional study of the current landscape of pediatric-capable mobile crisis capacity in the US as well as specific MCT staffing models that most effectively provide equitable youth crisis response are needed.

A safe place to be

"A safe place to be" involves a system to support youth and family that includes home-based and community-based stabilization services as well as acute care services.[51] Community-based and in-home behavioral health services should not be envisioned as an alternative to the crisis continuum but services "nested" within the continuum.[51] These services provide care coordination and support continuity of care through a community-based plan of care that is developed and implemented immediately after the crisis episode. Supports may include intensive in-home services, school-based and office-based services, family and youth peer support, as well as connection to natural supports within the youth's community. Although every priority should be made to provide a youth in crisis with stabilization within the home and community, sometimes, the safest immediate management of crisis is out-of-home stabilization.

Crisis Stabilization Units, Inpatient Care, and Alternative Models

For youth in crisis who were determined to require a higher level of care for psychiatric stabilization out of the community/home, the safest immediate location of care may be within a CSU or psychiatric inpatient setting. CSUs offer a safe and therapeutic alternative to EDs and inpatient units.[71] CSUs can provide psychiatric assessment, stabilization, observation, and short-term care.[72] Although not robustly studied in children, prior literature reports that for youth with suicidal ideation admitted to a CSU versus inpatient care, those on the CSU had significantly shorter stays with no differences in readmission rates or time to readmission compared to youth admitted to inpatient services.[73] Among adults in crisis, care in CSUs has been shown to reduce psychiatric admissions, decrease 30 day ED return visits, and increase 30 day follow-up visits.[74,75] Innovative models such as the living room model (a walk-in respite home-like environment), and the emergency psychiatric assessment, treatment, and healing unit (a stand-alone psychiatric emergency setting),[75,76] are not yet studied in children or youth, and therefore, efficacious specific customized approaches of CSU design for children and youth populations are currently unknown.

Inpatient psychiatric care can deliver vital services for youth with severe behavioral health symptoms.[77] However, inpatient stays can also come with significant burden to the youth including long periods of time disconnected from family and the community as well as separation from education or employment.[78] Various alternative models to inpatient care exist, with most utilizing community services and in-home services for youth in crisis. Examples of alternative models, which may be used in conjunction with each other and may include evidence-based practices, include intensive in-home treatment, intensive outpatient services, intensive care coordination using Wraparound, and, when the necessary services and supervision cannot be provided in the home, therapeutic foster care, and short-term residential interventions.[79-82] An international systematic review conducted in 2022 did not reveal sufficient data to recommend a specific alternative care model; however, in-home Multisystemic Therapy showed promise in improving a range of psychosocial parameters (including suicide attempts) with additional benefits to families (temporary adaptation and cohesion).[78] Additionally, although more than 40% of youth receiving in-home Multisystemic Therapy still required inpatient care, their length of stay was reduced compared to inpatient admission alone.[78] Given the increases in pediatric admissions for behavioral health conditions[83] as well as potential negative impact of inpatient admissions on youths,[78] further rigorous study of alternative treatment models compared to controls are urgently needed.

Postcrisis Services and Mental Health Follow-up

For the period after initial crisis stabilization, regardless of the level of mental health care needed, community-based and home-based services should have the capacity to provide care during the weeks after crisis stabilization.[51] Additionally, for youth who require inpatient psychiatric hospitalization, outpatient mental health follow-up within 7 days may be associated with a decreased suicide risk in the immediate postdischarge period and, therefore, is a core recommendation.[84,85] However, literature shows nearly half of youth discharged from the hospital are not receiving follow-up within a week, identifying opportunity to continue to build and enhance community, home, and outpatient services to meet the needs of this high-risk population.

INNOVATIONS
Psychiatric Urgent Care

A novel resource for risk assessment and determination of level of care for a youth in crisis is psychiatric urgent care. This emerging model provides access to short-term care and may include assessment, treatment (including initiation of medication-assisted treatment for substance use disorders), and referral to long-term services.[86] One study examined an urgent evaluation and care coordination service pilot that took referrals from schools for youth with safety concerns or behavior that severely affected school functioning, and found the model reduced pediatric ED visits.[87] Additionally, although not formally measured, the program received positive feedback from the schools involved.[87] A slightly different model is a bridge service that offers diversion from the ED, as well as immediate assessment, intervention, and short-term follow-up. One study of this service showed doubling of yearly volumes when incorporated within an academic center's proactive care delivery system.[88]

School-Based Care

Most youth spend more time in school than in any other setting outside of the home, making it an ideal place to screen, assess, and treat many behavioral health disorders. A systematic review and meta-analysis in 2021 showed that among the general population of youth, schools are the most common venue to receive mental health care.[89] Although assessment and treatment of behavioral health disorders is not an academic function per se, poor behavioral health can negatively impact academic outcomes.[90] An ideal comprehensive school mental health system includes educators, school-employed mental health professionals, and community and mental health providers, that collaborate across a multi-tiered system of support.[91,92] There are emerging data to suggest beneficial school-based mental health programs among all tiers from early identification through intervention.[92] New funding in 2023 through the US Department of Health and Human Services offers opportunity to create new and further expand school-based health centers throughout the US.[93] In the future, enhanced understanding of the specific successful school-based mental health center programs and partnerships with community mental health resources will likely strengthen the youth crisis continuum model.

Telehealth

States and communities are using telehealth to expand the delivery of crisis care to youth. Over 46 states have implemented telehealth initiatives such as child psychiatry access programs that provide training, technical assistance, and collaborative support to pediatric providers via immediate telephonic consultation, care coordination assistance, and professional education.[94,95] Several rural states have used technology platforms to remotely connect youth and families to crisis providers, avoiding interaction with law enforcement and diverting youth from ED and inpatient care. For example, Oklahoma has distributed more 30,000 Health Insurance Portability and Accountability Act (HIPAA) Health Insurance Portability and Accountability Act (HIPAA)-compliant electronic devices to individuals, schools, and first responders via its network of Certified Community Behavioral Health Clinics.[96] The devices immediately enable virtual communication with providers. Although not child-specific, a provider in the north-central and northeastern regions of the state had a 93.1% reduction in inpatient admissions after implementing tablet use.[96]

CONSIDERATIONS
Financial Sustainability

The financial sustainability of services across the crisis care continuum remains a challenge. Medicaid is now the single largest payer for behavioral health services[97] and the largest single insurer of children nationwide.[98] Even with the American Rescue Plan Act's time-limited Medicaid match enhancement,[99] Medicaid alone is unlikely to sustain the delivery of children's crisis services as reimbursement rates are lower than Medicare and commercial insurance.[89] Low reimbursement rates have constrained the physician provider pool[100]; similar constraints are likely among nonphysician mental health professionals delivering crisis services. Even commercial insurance is not optimal given that many payers do not cover crisis services, which limits funding for those youth that are covered by their caregiver's health insurance.

Funding sources that could be blended or braided to sustain service delivery to all youth, regardless of agency involvement or Medicaid eligibility,[101] include Medicaid, educational funds, child welfare dollars, state general funds, hospital community benefit dollars, and federal block grants.[102] Braided or blended funding involves coordination of 2 or more funding sources to support the total cost of a service by combining revenue from multiple funding streams into one "pot" to maximize flexibility across populations. A single entity or coordinated agency oversees all expenditures to ensure compliance with applicable statutes and regulations. However, these approaches can be administratively challenging, as some federal and state statutes prohibit blending of some funds, and braiding requires additional tracking and operational oversight.[102,103]

States and communities that have adopted a whole-population approach, which provides care for children regardless of payer source or agency involvement, have realized the most success in reducing an overreliance on acute care and institutional settings and in reducing child welfare and juvenile services caseloads.[104,105] Such states include New Jersey, which serves all children regardless of agency or payer involvement, and Massachusetts, which mandates state-regulated insurance coverage for crisis services.[106] Insurance mandates are complicated by the Employee Retirement Income Security Act of 1974, but given that nearly two-thirds of children are covered by a caregiver's commercial insurance plan,[107] states must consider that failure to adopt the whole-population approach burdens the public system while giving a free pass to the private one.

The challenge in which one agency bears costs that generate savings to an entirely different agency has been termed the "wrong pockets" problem.[108] Solving this "wrong pockets" problem and ensuring long-term sustainability typically requires incentivizing or mandating cross-agency collaboration to recapture and reinvest savings garnered by diversion from higher cost acute care, residential care, child welfare, and juvenile justice, to lower cost community-based crisis services.[102,109] States must consider how siloed agency budgets (or "pockets") could be aligned through mechanisms such as an interagency body[110,111] to maximize cross-sector flexibility.[102,112]

SUMMARY

This review describes existing crisis services for youth as well as essential components of an ideal youth-centered crisis response system, including the critical elements necessary to design, implement, study, and sustain the delivery of high-quality, developmentally appropriate services. As more US states develop and mature their respective 988 call centers and comprehensive response systems, youth-specific customization is necessary to ensure positive outcomes for youth, their families, and caregivers.

CLINICS CARE POINTS

- The ideal youth crisis continuum includes someone to talk to (crisis call and text lines), someone to respond (mobile crisis response), and a safe place to be (crisis stabilization) with a focus on keeping or returning youth to home- and community- based care as soon as it is safe and appropriate.

- Expanding innovations such as school-based behavioral health care and telehealth could extend reach of care to youth who live in settings with limited access to pediatric-specific supports.

- Creative funding models such as braided/blended funding or state-applied whole-population approaches are needed to ensure sustainability of youth crisis care.

ACKNOWLEDGEMENTS

The authors would like to acknowledge Deborah S. Harburger, MSW, for her review of the manuscript.

DISCLOSURE

The authors have no conflicts of interest relevant to this article to disclose. This article was completed without funding.

REFERENCES

1. Bitsko RH, Claussen AH, Lichstein J, et al. Mental health surveillance among children — United States, 2013–2019. MMWR Suppl 2022;71(2):1–42.
2. Keith P, Hawton K, Saunders KEA, et al. Self-harm and suicide in adolescents. Lancet 2012;379:2373–82.
3. Bridge JA, Ruch DA, Sheftall AH, et al. Youth suicide during the first year of the COVID-19 Pandemic. Pediatrics 2023;151(3).
4. Cummings JR, Wen H, Druss BG. Improving access to mental health services for youth in the United States. JAMA 2013;309(6):553–4.
5. Bastiampillai T, Sharfstein SS, Allison S. Increase in US suicide rates and the critical decline in psychiatric beds. JAMA, J Am Med Assoc 2016;316(24):2591–2.
6. Satiani A, Niedermier J, Satiani B, et al. Projected workforce of psychiatrists in the United States: A population analysis. Psychiatr Serv 2018;69(6):710–3.
7. American Academy of Child & Adolescent Psychiatry. Workforce issues. 2019. Available at: https://www.aacap.org/aacap/resources_for_primary_care/workforce_issues.aspx#:~:text=There%20are%20approximately%208%2C300%20practicing,a%20child%20and%20adolescent%20psychiatrist. [Accessed 4 February 2024].
8. Whitney DG, Peterson MD. US national and state-level prevalence of mental health disorders and disparities of mental health care use in children. JAMA Pediatr 2019;173(4):389–91.
9. Hoffmann JA, Attridge MM, Carroll MS, et al. Association of youth suicides and county-level mental health professional shortage areas in the US. JAMA Pediatr 2023;177(1):71–80.
10. Schnitzer PG, Dykstra H, Collier A. The COVID-19 pandemic and youth suicide: 2020-2021. Pediatrics 2023;151(3).
11. Racine N, McArthur BA, Cooke JE, et al. Global prevalence of depressive and anxiety symptoms in children and adolescents during COVID-19: a meta-analysis. JAMA Pediatr 2021;175(11):1142–50.
12. Arakelyan M, Emond JA, Leyenaar JAK. Suicide and self-harm in youth presenting to a us rural hospital during COVID-19. Hosp Pediatr 2022;12(10):E336–42.
13. Krass P, Dalton E, Doupnik SK, et al. US pediatric emergency department visits for mental health conditions during the COVID-19 pandemic. JAMA Netw Open 2021;4(4):e218533.

14. American Academy of Pediatrics American Academy of Child and Adolescent Psychiatry & Children's Hospital Association. Declaration of a national emergency in child and adolescent mental health. 2021. Accessed February 4, 2024.
15. Office of the Surgeon General (OSG). Protecting youth mental health: the U.S. Surgeon General's Advisory [Internet]. Washington (DC): US Department of Health and Human Services; 2021. Available at: https://www.ncbi.nlm.nih.gov/books/NBK575984/. [Accessed 4 February 2024].
16. Bommersbach TJ, Mckean AJ, Olfson M, et al. National trends in mental health-related emergency department visits among youth, 2011-2020. JAMA 2023; 329(17):1469–77.
17. Leith T, Brieger K, Malas N, et al. Increased prevalence and severity of psychiatric illness in hospitalized youth during COVID-19. Clin Child Psychol Psychiatry 2022;27(3):804–12.
18. Hoffmann JA, Stack AM, Monuteaux MC, et al. Factors associated with boarding and length of stay for pediatric mental health emergency visits. AJEM (Am J Emerg Med) 2019;37(10):1829–35.
19. McEnany FB, Ojugbele O, Doherty JR, et al. Pediatric Mental Health Boarding. Pediatrics 2020;146(4):e20201174.
20. Foster AA, Sundberg M, Williams DN, et al. Emergency department staff perceptions about the care of children with mental health conditions. Gen Hosp Psychiatry 2021;73:78–83.
21. Wolff JC, Maron M, Chou T, et al. Experiences of child and adolescent psychiatric patients boarding in the emergency department from staff perspectives: patient journey mapping. Adm Policy Ment Health 2023;50(3):417–26.
22. Bakhsh HT, Perona SJ, Shields WA, et al. Medication errors in psychiatric patients boarded in the emergency department. Int J Risk Saf Med 2014;26(4): 191–8.
23. Sethuraman U, Kannikeswaran N, Farooqi A, et al. Antipsychiatric medication errors in children boarded in a pediatric emergency department. Pediatr Emerg Care 2021;37(9):e358–542.
24. Kulstad EB, Sikka R, Sweis RT, et al. ED overcrowding is associated with an increased frequency of medication errors. AJEM (Am J Emerg Med) 2010; 28(3):304–9.
25. Nash KA, Zima BT, Rothenberg C, et al. Prolonged emergency department length of stay for US pediatric mental health visits (2005–2015). Pediatrics 2021;147(5). e2020030692.
26. Stroul B, Blau G, Friedman R. Updating the system of care concept and philosophy. Washington, DC: Georgetown University Center for Child and Human Development, National Technical Assistance Center for Children's Mental Health; 2010.
27. Stroul BA, Blau GM, Larsen J. The evolution of the system of care approach. Baltimore: The Institute for Innovation and Implementation, School of Social Work, University of Maryland; 2021.
28. Lindsey M, Sheftall A, Xiao Y, et al. Trends of suicidal behaviors among high school students in the United States: 1991–2017. Pediatrics 2019;144(5).
29. Raifman J, Charlton BM, Arrington-Sanders R, et al. Sexual orientation and suicide attempt disparities among US adolescents: 2009-2017. Pediatrics 2020; 145(3).
30. Williams DR. Stress and the mental health of populations of color: advancing our understanding of race-related stressors. J Health Soc Behav 2018;59(4): 466–85.

31. Trent M, Dooley DG, Dougé J, et al. The impact of racism on child and adolescent health. Pediatrics 2019;144(2).

32. Stephens TN. Distinguishing racism, not race, as a risk factor for child welfare involvement: reclaiming the familial and cultural strengths in the lived experiences of child welfare-affected parents of color. Genealogy 2021;5(1):11.

33. Bridge JA, Horowitz LM, Fontanella CA, et al. Age-related racial disparity in suicide rates among US Youths From 2001 Through 2015. JAMA Pediatr 2018; 172(7):696–7.

34. Sheftall AH, Vakil F, Ruch DA, et al. Black youth suicide: investigation of current trends and precipitating circumstances. J Am Acad Child Adolesc Psychiatry 2022;61(5):662–75.

35. Fontanella CA, Hiance-Steelesmith DL, Phillips GS, et al. Widening rural-urban disparities in youth suicides, United States, 1996-2010. JAMA Pediatr 2015; 169(5):466–73.

36. Graves JM, Abshire DA, MacKelprang JL, et al. Association of Rurality with Availability of Youth Mental Health Facilities with Suicide Prevention Services in the US. JAMA Netw Open 2020;3(10).

37. Centers for Disease Control and Prevention WISQARS fatal injury reports, national, regional, and state, 1981-2018. https://webappa.cdc.gov/sasweb/ncipc/mortrate.html-Accessed June 24, 2024.

38. Kelleher KJ, Gardner W. Out of sight, out of mind — behavioral and developmental care for rural children. N Engl J Med 2017;376(14):1301–3.

39. Luk JW, Goldstein RB, Yu J, et al. Sexual minority status and age of onset of adolescent suicide ideation and behavior. Pediatrics 2021;148(4).

40. Rhoades H, Rusow JA, Bond D, et al. Homelessness, mental health and suicidality among LGBTQ youth accessing crisis services. Child Psychiatry Hum Dev 2018;49(4):643–51.

41. Katz CC, Gopalan G, Wall E, et al. Screening and assessment of suicidal behavior in transition-age youth with foster care involvement. Child Adolesc Soc Work J 2023;13:1–13.

42. McMillen JC, Zima BT, Scott LD, Auslander WF, Munson MR, Ollie MT, Spitznagel EL. Prevalence of psychiatric disorders among older youths in the foster care system. Journal of teh American Academy of Child and Adolescent Psychiatry. 2005;44(1):88–95.

43. Rivera M, Sullivan R. Rethinking child welfare to keep families safe and together: effective housing-based supports to reduce child trauma, maltreatment recidivism, and re-entry to foster care. Child Welfare 2015;94(4):185–204.

44. Kids Count Data Center. Children entering foster care by age in United States. 2023. Available at: https://datacenter.aecf.org/data/tables/6244-children-in-foster-care-by-age-group#detailed/1/any/false/2048574,1729,37,871,870,573,869,36,868/1889,2616,2617,2618,2619,122/12988,12989. [Accessed 4 February 2024].

45. Larson S, Neidorf J, Pettingell S, et al. Long-term supports and services for persons with intellectual or developmental disabilities: Status and trends through 2019. Minneapolis: University of Minnesota, Institute on Community Integration; 2022.

46. Walensky RP, Bunnell R, Kent CK, et al. Prevalence and characteristics of autism spectrum disorder among children aged 8 years-autism and developmental disabilities monitoring network, 11 Sites, United States, 2020. 2020. MMWR Surveill Summ 2023;72(SS722):4–14.

47. Lai MC, Kassee C, Besney R, et al. Prevalence of co-occurring mental health diagnoses in the autism population: a systematic review and meta-analysis. Lancet Psychiatr 2019;6(10):819–29.

48. Bloom SR, Kuhlthau K, Van Cleave J, et al. Health care transition for youth with special health care needs. J Adolesc Health 2012;51(3):213–9.

49. Kurtz PF, Leoni M, Hagopian LP. Behavioral approaches to assessment and early intervention for severe problem behavior in intellectual and developmental disabilities. Pediatr Clin North Am 2020;67(3):499–511.

50. Substance Abuse and Mental Health Services Administration. National Guidelines for Child and Youth Behavioral Health Crisis Care. Publication No. PEP22-01-02-001 Rockville, MD: Substance Abuse and Mental Health Services Administration. 2022. Available at: https://www.samhsa.gov/data/.

51. Schober M, Harburger DS, Sulzbach D, et al. A safe place to Be: crisis stabilization services and other supports for children and youth. Technical assistance collaborative Paper No. 4. Alexandria, VA: National Association of State Mental Health Program Directors; 2022.

52. Mathieu SL, Uddin R, Brady M, et al. Systematic review: the state of research into youth helplines. J Am Acad Child Adolesc Psychiatry 2021;60(10): 1190–233.

53. Fix RL, Bandara S, Fallin MD, et al. Creating comprehensive crisis response systems: an opportunity to build on the promise of 988. Community Ment Health J 2023;59(2):205–8.

54. Hoover S, Bostic J. Improving the child and adolescent crisis system: Shifting from a 9-1-1 to a 9-8-8 Paradigm. Alexandria, VA: National Association of State Mental Health Program Directors; 2020.

55. Brooks Holliday S, Matthews S, Bialas A, et al. A Qualitative Investigation of Preparedness for the Launch of 988: Implications for the Continuum of Emergency Mental Health Care. Adm Policy Ment Health 2023;50(4):616–29.

56. National Academy for State Health Policy. State Legislation to Fund and Implement the 988 Suicide and Crisis Lifeline. 2023. Available at: https://nashp.org/state-tracker/state-legislation-to-fund-and-implement-988-for-the-national-suicide-prevention-lifeline/. [Accessed 4 February 2024].

57. Lenhart A, Ling R, Campbell S, et al. Teens and Mobile Phones. 2010. Accessed February 4, 2024.

58. Harris BR. Helplines for mental health support: perspectives of New York state college students and implications for promotion and implementation of 988. Community Ment Health J 2024;60(1):191–9.

59. Gould MS, Chowdhury S, Lake AM, et al. National Suicide Prevention Lifeline crisis chat interventions: Evaluation of chatters' perceptions of effectiveness. Suicide Life Threat Behav 2021;51(6):1126–37.

60. Pisani AR, Gould MS, Gallo C, et al. Individuals who text crisis text line: Key characteristics and opportunities for suicide prevention. Suicide Life Threat Behav 2022;52(3):567–82.

61. Mark T, Misra S, Howard J, et al. Inpatient Bed Tracking: State Responses to Need for Inpatient Care. 2019. Available at: https://aspe.hhs.gov/reports/inpatient-bed-tracking-state-responses-need-inpatient-care-0. [Accessed 4 February 2024].

62. Compton MT, Bakeman R, Broussard B, et al. The police-based Crisis Intervention Team (CIT) model: II. Effects on level of force and resolution, referral and arrest. Psychiatr Serv 2014;65(4):523–9.

63. Balfour ME, Hahn Stephenson A, Delany-Brumsey A, et al. Cops, Clinicians, or Both? Collaborative Approaches to Responding to Behavioral Health Emergencies. Psychiatr Serv 2022;73(6):658–69.

64. Fendrich M, Ives M, Kurz B, et al. Impact of mobile crisis services on emergency department use among youths with behavioral health service needs. Psychiatr Serv 2019;70(10):881–7.

65. Lui JHL, Chen BC, Benson LA, Lin Ruiz A, Lau AS. Inpatient Care Utilization Following Mobile Crisis Response Encounters Among Racial/Ethnic Minoritized Youth. Journal of the American Academy of Child and Adolescent Psychiatry 2024;63(7):720–32. https://doi.org/10.1016/j.jaac.2023.06.021.

66. Oblath R, Herrera CN, Were LPO, et al. Long-Term Trends in Psychiatric Emergency Services Delivered by the Boston Emergency Services Team. Community Ment Health J 2023;59(2):370–80.

67. Department of Health & Human Services. Centers for Medicare & Medicaid Services. Medicaid Guidance on the Scope of and Payments for Qualifying Community-Based Mobile Crisis Intervention Services. 2021. Available at: https://www.medicaid.gov/sites/default/files/2021-12/sho21008.pdf. [Accessed 4 February 2024].

68. Ojeda VD, Munson MR, Jones N, et al. The Availability of Peer Support and Disparities in Outpatient Mental Health Service Use Among Minority Youth with Serious Mental Illness. Adm Pol Ment Health 2021;48(2):290–8.

69. King AJ, Simmons MB. "The Best of Both Worlds": Experiences of young people attending groups co-facilitated by peer workers and clinicians in a youth mental health service. Early Interv Psychiatry 2023;17(1):65–75.

70. Jackson DB, Fahmy C, Vaughn MG, et al. Police Stops Among At-Risk Youth: Repercussions for Mental Health. J Adolesc Health 2019;65(5):627–32.

71. Substance Abuse and Mental Health Services Administration. Crisis services: effectiveness, cost-effectiveness, and funding Strategies. HHS Publication No. (SMA)-14-4848. Rockville, MD: Substance Abuse and Mental Health Services Administration; 2014.

72. Saxon Verletta. Behavioral Health Crisis Stabilization Centers: A New Normal. Journal of Mental Health and Clinical Psychology 2018;2:23–6.

73. Otterson SE, Fristad MA, McBee-Strayer S, et al. Length of stay and readmission data for adolescents psychiatrically treated on a youth crisis stabilization unit versus a traditional inpatient unit. Evid Based Pract Child Adolesc Ment Health 2021;6(4):484–9.

74. Anderson K, Goldsmith LP, Lomani J, et al. Short-stay crisis units for mental health patients on crisis care pathways: systematic review and meta-analysis. BJPsych Open 2022;8(4).

75. Kim AK, Vakkalanka JP, Van Heukelom P, et al. Emergency psychiatric assessment, treatment, and healing (EmPATH) unit decreases hospital admission for patients presenting with suicidal ideation in rural America. Acad Emerg Med 2022;29(2):142–9.

76. Heyland M, Emery C, Shattell M. The living room, a community crisis respite program: offering people in crisis an alternative to emergency departments. Glob J Community Psychol Pract 2013;4(3):1–8. Retrieved 4/04/2023, from (Available at: http://www.gjcpp.org/.

77. Green J, Jacobs B, Beecham J, et al. Inpatient treatment in child and adolescent psychiatry - A prospective study of health gain and costs. J Child Psychol Psychiatry 2007;48(12):1259–67.

78. Clisu DA, Layther I, Dover D, et al. Alternatives to mental health admissions for children and adolescents experiencing mental health crises: A systematic review of the literature. Clin Child Psychol Psychiatry 2022;27(1):35–60.

79. Shepperd S, Doll H, Gowers S, et al. Alternatives to inpatient mental health care for children and young people. Cochrane Database Syst Rev 2009;(2): CD006410.

80. Kwok KHR, Yuan SNV, Ougrin D. Review: Alternatives to inpatient care for children and adolescents with mental health disorders. Child Adolesc Ment Health 2016;21(1):3–10.

81. Olson JR, Benjamin PH, Azman AA, Kellogg MA, Pullmann MD, Suter JC, Bruns EJ. Systematic Review and Meta-analysis: Effectiveness of Wraparound Care Coordination for Children and Adolescents. Journal of the American Academy of Child and Adolescent Psychiatry 2021;60(11):1353–66. https://doi.org/10.1016/j.jaac.2021.02.022.

82. Tsai D. Leveraging medicaid, CHIP, and Other Federal Programs in the Delivery of Behavioral Health Services for Children and Youth. CMCS Informational Bulletin. 2022. Access June 25, 2024. https://www.medicaid.gov/federal-policy-guidance/downloads/bhccib08182022.pdf

83. Torio CM, Encinosa W, Berdahl T, et al. Annual report on health care for children and youth in the United States: national estimates of cost, utilization and expenditures for children with mental health conditions. Acad Pediatr 2015;15:19–35.

84. Fontanella CA, Warner LA, Steelesmith DL, et al. Association of timely outpatient mental health services for youths after psychiatric hospitalization with risk of death by suicide. JAMA Netw Open 2020;3(8):E2012887.

85. Centers for Medicare & Medicaid Services. Children's health care quality measures: core set of children's health care quality measures. Available at: https://www.medicaid.gov/medicaid/quality-of-care/performance-measurement/adult-and-child-health-care-quality-measures/childrens-health-care-quality-measures/index.html. [Accessed 8 February 2024].

86. Sunderji N, Tan De Bibiana J, Stergiopoulos V. Urgent psychiatric services: a scoping review. Can J Psychiatry 2015;60(9):393–402.

87. Alvarado G, Hegg L, Rhodes K. Improving psychiatric access for students in crisis: An alternative to the emergency department. Psychiatr Serv 2020;71(8): 864–7.

88. Sorter M, Stark LJ, Glauser T, et al. Addressing the pediatric mental health crisis: moving from a reactive to a proactive system of care. J Pediatr 2024;265: 113479.

89. Duong MT, Bruns EJ, Lee K, et al. Rates of Mental Health Service Utilization by Children and Adolescents in Schools and Other Common Service Settings: A Systematic Review and Meta-Analysis. Adm Policy Ment Health 2021;48(3): 420–39.

90. Kase C, Hoover S, Boyd G, et al. Educational Outcomes Associated With School Behavioral Health Interventions: A Review of the Literature. J Sch Health 2017; 87(7):554–62.

91. The National Center for School Mental Health and National Association of School Psychologists. Effective School-Community Partnerships to Support School Mental Health. Accessed June 24, 2024. https://schoolmentalhealth.org/resources/

92. Hoover S, Bostic J. Schools As a Vital Component of the Child and Adoelescent Mental Health System. Psychiatric Services. 2021 Jan 1; 72 (1):37-48.

93. U.S. Department of Health and Human Services Health Resources and Services Administration. The Biden-Harris Administration Invests $55 Million in Expanding Access to Youth Mental Health Care. September 25, 2023. Accesss June 24, 2024. https://www.hrsa.gov/about/news/press-release/fy-2023-youth-mental-health-care.

94. National Network of Child Psychiatry Access Programs. Child Psychiatry Access Programs in the United States. Map Revised 03.14.23. Available at: https://www.nncpap.org/map. [Accessed 4 February 2024].

95. Campo B. iPads help law enforcement and others connect people in crisis to mental health resources. 2023. Available at: https://oklahoma.gov/odmhsas/about/public-information/press-releases-and-other-news/2023/ipads-help-law-enforcement—others-connect-people-in-crisis-to-.html. [Accessed 4 February 2024].

96. Health Resources and Services Administration Maternal & Child Health. Pediatric Mental Health Care Access Program (PMHCA): Improving Behavioral Health Services. Last Revised March 2024. Accessed June 20, 2024. https://mchb.hrsa.gov/programs-impact/programs/pediatric-mental-health-care-access.

97. Breslau J, Han B, Lai J, et al. Impact of the affordable care act medicaid expansion on utilization of mental health care. Med Care 2020;58(9):757–62.

98. Brooks-Lasure C, Tsai D. A Strategic Vision for Medicaid and The Children's Health Insurance Program (CHIP). 2021. Available at: https://www.healthaffairs.org/content/forefront/strategic-vision-medicaid-and-children-s-health-insurance-program-chip. [Accessed 4 February 2024].

99. American Rescue Plan Act of 2021. House of Representatives- Budget. H.R. 1319. 117-2. 2021. Available at: https://www.congress.gov/bill/117th-congress/house-bill/1319/text.

100. Alexander D, Schnell M. The Impacts of Physician Payments on Patient Access, Use, and Health. 2019.

101. Clary A, Riley T. Braiding & Blending Funding Streams to Meet the Health-Related Social Needs of Low-Income Persons: Considerations for State Health Policymakers. 2016. Available at: https://housingis.org/sites/default/files/BraidingBlendingNASHP.pdf. [Accessed 4 February 2024].

102. Harburger DS, Pires SA, Schober MA. Sustainable financing to support children & families: Medicaid and other fiscal, funding, and financing challenges and opportunities, In: Denby-Brinson R, Ingram C. Child and family-serving systems: A compendium of policy and practice (Volume I: Evolution of protecting, strengthening, and sustaining children and families), 2022, CWLA Press.

103. US Government Accountability Office.Child Care: Information on Integrating Early Care and Education Funding, GAO-16-775R Child Care. 2016. Available at: https://eric.ed.gov/?id=ED572236. [Accessed 4 February 2024].

104. Federal Communications Commissions. 2020 Broadband Deployment Report. 2020. Available at: https://docs.fcc.gov/public/attachments/FCC-20-50A1.pdf. [Accessed 4 February 2024].

105. Substance Abuse and Mental Health Services Administration. The Comprehensive Community Mental Health Services for Children with Serious Emotional Disturbances Program, Report to Congress. 2015. Available at: https://store.samhsa.gov/product/comprehensive-community-mental-health-services-children-serious-emotional-disturbances. [Accessed 4 February 2024].

106. Anderson G, Mikula J. Access to Services to Treat Child-Adolescent Mental Health Disorders. https://www.mass.gov/doc/bulletin-2018-07-access-to-services-to-treat-child-adolescent-mental-health-disorders-issued/download.

107. Keisler-Starkey K, Bunch L. Health Insurance Coverage in the United States: 2021. 2022. Available at: https://www.census.gov/library/publications/2022/demo/p60-278.html. [Accessed 8 February 2024].

108. Roman JK. Solving the wrong pockets problem. 2015. Available at: https://pfs.urban.org/system/files/2000427-solving-the-wrong-pockets-problem.pdf. [Accessed 4 February 2024].

109. Stroul B, Pires S, Boyce S, et al. Return on investment in systems of care for children with behavioral health challenges. Washington, DC: Georgetown University Center for Child and Human Development, National Technical Assistance Center for Children's Mental Health; 2014.

110. Tai MH, Lee B, Onukwugha E, et al. Impact of a care management entity on use of psychiatric services among youths with severe mental or behavioral disorders. Psychiatr Serv 2018;69(11):1167–74.

111. Sulzbach D, Wilkness S, Virgo K, et al. The Role of Children's Cabinets in Advancing and Sustaining Systems of Care. Training Institutes. Baltimore, Maryland July 25-28, 2018. Available at: https://www.nmlegis.gov/handouts/LHHS%20082218%20Item%2011%20public%20comment_Monica%20Miura_Role_of_Children%27s_Cabinets_in_SOCs.pdf. [Accessed 4 February 2024].

112. Butlet S. How "Wong Pockets" Hurt Health. JAMA Forum Archive. Published online August 22, 2018. Accessed June 20, 2024. https://jamanetwork.com/channels/health-forum/fullarticle/2760141.

Moving?

Make sure your subscription moves with you!

To notify us of your new address, find your **Clinics Account Number** (located on your mailing label above your name), and contact customer service at:

Email: journalscustomerservice-usa@elsevier.com

800-654-2452 (subscribers in the U.S. & Canada)
314-447-8871 (subscribers outside of the U.S. & Canada)

Fax number: 314-447-8029

**Elsevier Health Sciences Division
Subscription Customer Service
3251 Riverport Lane
Maryland Heights, MO 63043**

*To ensure uninterrupted delivery of your subscription, please notify us at least 4 weeks in advance of move.

Printed and bound by CPI Group (UK) Ltd, Croydon, CR0 4YY

08/05/2025

01864724-0011